Recent Results in Cancer Research 188

Hans-Jörg Senn • Florian Otto
(Editors)

Clinical Cancer Prevention

Springer

Editors
Prof. Hans-Jörg Senn
Tumor- and Breast-Center ZeTuP
Rorschacherstrasse 150
9006 St. Gallen, Switzerland
hjsenn@sg.zetup.ch

Prof. Dr. med. Florian Otto
Tumor- and Breast-Center ZeTuP
Rorschacherstrasse 150
9006 St. Gallen, Switzerland
fotto@sg.zetup.ch

ISBN 978-3-642-10856-3 e-ISBN 978-3-642-10858-7
DOI 10.1007/978-3-642-10858-7
Springer Heidelberg Dordrecht London New York

Library of Congress Control Number: 2010933082

Cover design: eStudio Calamar Figueres/Berlin

Printed on acid-free paper

Springer is part of Springer Science+Business Media (www.springer.com)

Contents

1 **Allocating Cancer-Directed Expenditures: Tensions Between Prevention, Early Detection and Treatment is Unnecessary** 1
Bruce E. Hillner and Thomas J. Smith

1.1 Introduction 1
1.2 Our Life Expectancy and Cancer Success Stories 2
1.3 No Cure in Sight: Costs of Drugs, Gadgets, Genomics and Technology 2
1.4 Bending the Cancer Cost Curve 5
1.5 Conclusion 8
References 8

2 **Lessons Learned from Prevention Programs: Different Endpoints Should Be Used in Secondary and Tertiary Prevention** 11
Franz Porzsolt

2.1 Introduction 11
2.2 Methods 12
2.3 Results 13
2.3.1 Traditional Outcomes of Treatment and of Prevention Programs 13
2.3.2 Proposal for the Evaluation of Prevention Programs 15
2.4 Discussion 16
2.4.1 The Risk of Interpretation in Prevention Programs 16
2.4.2 The Resulting Need for Evaluation of Preventive Medicine 17
2.4.3 Recommendations for Future Preventive Research 18
References 18

3 Biomarkers for Early Detection and as Surrogate Endpoints in Cancer Prevention Trials: Issues and Opportunities 21
Barbara K. Dunn, Karin Jegalian, and Peter Greenwald

Abbreviations 21
3.1 Biomarkers: What They Are and How They Are Applied 23
3.1.1 Screening Biomarkers for Early Detection 23
3.1.2 Biomarkers as Surrogate Endpoints in Cancer Prevention Trials 26
3.2 Breast Precancer and Cancer Prevention 28
3.2.1 Ductal Carcinoma In situ 30
3.2.2 Tissue Stroma and Mammographic Density 31
3.2.3 Biomarkers, ER-Positive Breast Cancer, and Breast Cancer Prevention Trials 31
3.2.4 Biomarkers and Estrogen Receptor-Negative Breast Cancers 33
3.2.5 Access to Breast Tissue for Biomarker Evaluation 33
3.2.6 Biomarkers in Phase 2 Chemoprevention Trials 34
3.3 Prostate Cancer Prevention 35
3.3.1 PSA Screening and Early Detection of Prostate Cancer 35
3.3.2 Phase 3 Prostate Cancer Prevention Trials 35
3.3.3 Discovery of New Biomarkers for Early Detection of Prostate Cancer 36
3.4 Colorectal Cancer Prevention 37
3.5 Lung Cancer Prevention 38
3.5.1 Molecular Markers for Early Detection and Prognosis 39
3.5.2 Treating Nicotine Addiction 40
3.5.3 Fluorescence Bronchoscopy 40
3.6 Conclusions 40
References 40

4 Targeting Polyamines and Inflammation for Cancer Prevention 49
Naveen Babbar and Eugene W. Gerner

4.1 Introduction 50
4.2 Polyamines, Inflammation, and Cancer 50
4.2.1 Polyamine Metabolism 50
4.2.2 Polyamines and Cancer 52
4.3 Roles of Inflammation and Polyamines in Prostate Cancer 53
4.3.1 Polyamines and Prostate Cancer 53
4.3.2 Polyamines, Inflammation, and Prostate Cancer 53
4.3.3 Targeting Polyamines and Inflammation in Prostate Cancer 54
4.4 Roles of Inflammation and Polyamines in Colon Cancer 55
4.4.1 Polyamines and Colon Cancer 55
4.4.2 Polyamines, Inflammation, and Colon Cancer 56
4.4.3 Targeting Polyamines and Inflammation in Colon Cancer 56

4.5 Roles of Inflammation and Polyamines in Other Cancers 59
4.6 Conclusions 60
References 60

5 Thinking About the Role (Largely Ignored) of Heavy Metals in Cancer Prevention: Hexavalent Chromium and Melanoma as a Case in Point 65
Frank L. Meyskens and Sun Yang

5.1 Background 65
5.1.1 The Evolution of the Idea 65
5.1.2 Substances That Bind Melanin 66
5.2 Major Risk Factors for Cutaneous Melanoma 67
5.2.1 Epidemiology 67
5.3 Metals 69
5.3.1 Chemistry and Genetic Damage 69
5.3.2 Chromium Chemistry 69
5.3.3 Upregulation of Metallothioneins (MTs) 70
5.3.4 Some Preliminary Experimental Data 70
5.4 Future Prospects 72
References 72

6 Hepatitis B Virus and Cancer Prevention 75
Mei-Hwei Chang

6.1 Infection and Cancer 75
6.2 Disease Burden of Liver Cancer 77
6.3 Hepatitis B Virus Infection and Hepatocellular Carcinoma 77
6.4 Cancer Prevention Against Hepatocellular Carcinoma 78
6.5 Hepatitis B Vaccination Program 79
6.6 Effective Reduction of Chronic HBV Infection by Universal Hepatitis B Immunization 79
6.7 The Effect on Liver Cancer Prevention by Vaccination 80
6.8 Problems and Strategies of Successful HCC Prevention by Hepatitis B Vaccination 81
6.9 Implications and Future Prospects 81
References 82

7 Chemoprevention of Hepatocellular Carcinoma in Chronic Hepatitis C 85
Timothy R. Morgan

7.1 Hepatitis C 85
7.2 Hepatocellular Carcinoma 86
7.3 Prevention of Hepatocellular Carcinoma 87
7.3.1 Curative Treatment 87

7.3.2 Treatments That Suppress Hepatitis C Virus 88
7.3.3 Noncurative Chemoprevention 88
7.3.4 Prospective Randomized Trials:
Carotenoids and Phytochemicals 88
7.3.5 Secondary Chemoprevention of HCC 89
7.3.6 Nonrandomized, Uncontrolled and/or
Retrospective Clinical Trials 90
7.3.7 Epidemiologic Studies 91
7.3.8 Drugs Used to Treat Hepatocellular Carcinoma 92
7.3.9 Prevention of Hepatocellular Carcinoma in Cell Lines
and Animal Models 92
7.3.10 Phase II Trial of *S*-Adenosylmethionine
in Hepatitis C Cirrhosis 94
7.4 Conclusions 97
References 97

8 Nutritional Aspects of Primary Prostate Cancer Prevention 101
Hans-Peter Schmid, Claus Fischer, Daniel S. Engeler,
Marcelo L. Bendhack, and Bernd J. Schmitz-Dräger

8.1 Introduction 101
8.2 Dietary/Nutritional Factors 102
8.2.1 Dietary Fat 102
8.2.2 Obesity 102
8.2.3 Micronutrients 102
8.2.4 Vitamins 103
8.2.5 Minerals 103
8.2.6 Phytoestrogens 104
8.2.7 Diabetes Mellitus 104
8.3 American Cancer Society (ACS) Guideline 105
8.3.1 A: Try to Maintain a Healthy Weight 105
8.3.2 B: Take Regular Physical Exercise 105
8.3.3 C: Maintain a Healthy Diet with a Focus
on Fruit and Vegetables 105
8.3.4 D: Reduce Alcohol Intake 105
8.4 Conclusions 106
References 106

9 Prostate Cancer Prevention with 5 Alpha-Reductase Inhibitors 109
Dipen J. Parekh

9.1 Rationale for the Chemoprevention of Prostate Cancer 109
9.2 The Prostate Cancer Prevention Trial 110
9.3 Pathologic Characteristics of the Cancers in
the Prostate Cancer Prevention Trial 110

9.4 Finasteride Increases Sensitivity of Prostate-Specific Antigen, Digital Rectal Examination and Biopsy Detection for Prostate Cancer. 111
9.4.1 Decreased Prostate Volume with Finasteride Increases Cancer Detection. 112
9.5 Side Effects of Finasteride 113
9.6 Conclusion 113
References. 113

10 Hormone Replacement Therapy and Breast Cancer. 115
Anthony Howell and Gareth D. Evans

10.1 Background. 115
10.2 HRT Use in Women Diagnosed with Breast Cancer 116
10.2.1 Observational Studies 116
10.2.2 Randomised Trials 117
10.2.3 Effects of Withdrawal of HRT in Women with Breast Cancer. 117
10.3 HRT and Risk of Breast Cancer 118
10.3.1 Observational Studies 118
10.3.2 Randomised Studies 118
10.3.3 Withdrawal of HRT in Women Without Breast Cancer 119
10.3.4 Summary. 119
10.4 HRT After Oophorectomy in Women Less Than 50 Years of Age 119
10.4.1 Observational Studies. 120
10.5 Coronary Heart Disease 120
10.6 Potential Biological Explanations. 121
10.7 Conclusions. 122
References. 122

11 Physical Activity and Breast Cancer: Review of the Epidemiologic Evidence and Biologic Mechanisms. 125
Christine M. Friedenreich

11.1 Epidemiologic Evidence. 126
11.1.1 Background. 126
11.1.2 Methodologic Issues in Studies of Physical Activity and Cancer 126
11.1.3 Overall Associations Between Physical Activity and Breast Cancer Risk. 126
11.1.4 Type, Dose, and Timing of Activity 126
11.1.5 Population Subgroups. 128
11.1.6 Summary of Epidemiologic Findings. 131
11.2 Biologic Mechanisms 132
11.2.1 Adiposity. 132
11.2.2 Sex Hormones. 132

11.2.3 Insulin-Related Factors 134
11.2.4 Adipokines and Inflammation 134
11.2.5 Other Mechanisms 135
11.3 Conclusion 135
References 136

12 Prevention of Breast Cancer by Newer SERMs in the Future 141
Trevor Powles

12.1 Introduction 141
12.2 Arzoxifene 142
12.3 Lasofoxifene 142
12.4 Discussion 143
12.5 Conclusions 144
References 144

13 Chemoprevention of Hormone Receptor-Negative Breast Cancer: New Approaches Needed 147
Iván P. Uray and Powel H. Brown

13.1 Introduction 148
13.2 Endocrine Preventive Agents 148
13.3 Selective Estrogen Receptor Modulators 148
13.4 Aromatase Inhibitors 151
13.5 New Strategies to Prevent Hormone-Independent Breast Cancer 152
13.5.1 PARP Inhibitors 152
13.6 Cell Growth Inhibitors 153
13.6.1 Statins 153
13.6.2 Metformin 153
13.6.3 Retinoids 154
13.6.4 PPAR Agonists 156
13.6.5 COX-2 Inhibitors 156
13.6.6 Tyrosine Kinase Inhibitors 157
13.6.7 The IGF System 158
13.6.8 Conclusions and Future Directions 158
References 159

Allocating Cancer-Directed Expenditures: Tensions Between Prevention, Early Detection and Treatment is Unnecessary

1

Bruce E. Hillner and Thomas J. Smith

Abstract In most countries, the allocation of financial resources for cancer prevention, early detection, and treatment come from different nonrelated "silos." Primary prevention benefits have the greatest economic return since the cancer benefits are intertwined with other major health conditions. Smoking alone accounts for about one-third cancer deaths. In most affluent countries, vaccines for selected viral caused cancers are (wisely) widely available if not optimally utilized. Estimating the additional cancer burden from obesity is still evolving. Age-targeted, less frequent but higher rates of participation in early detection of cervical, breast, and colorectal cancer will likely be prudent expenditures.

The last 20 years in high-income countries, there has seen an explosion in demand and the costs of cancer drug or biologic therapy, a modest growth in some forms of radiation, yet minimal or declining surgical costs for primary disease control. Expenditures for cancer drugs are now the world leader of any medication category. While a few have truly led to marked benefits, all have been priced at levels that strain or break budgets. We comment on ten steps or principles that can be applied in most countries that can meaningfully reduce cancer care costs with minimal impact on survival and maintain or enhance quality of patient's life especially with advanced disease. We emphasize limiting systemic therapies for metastatic disease to fully ambulatory patients, those who previously responded to therapy, and earlier initiation of palliative care. Changing behaviors, incentives, expectations, and the framing of treatment effects are necessary to "bend" the current unrelenting cancer care cost curve.

1.1 Introduction

To paraphase Dickens, it is the best and worst of times depending on one's perspective when considering the societal impact of cancer. The costs of cancer treatment especially for advanced or recurrent disease are rapidly and persistently increasing. The symposium directors have

B.E. Hillner (✉) and T.J. Smith
Department of Internal Medicine and the Massey Cancer Center, Virginia Commonwealth University, 1101 E. Marshall St. Room 7013, Richmond, VA 23298-0170, USA
e-mail: hillner@vcu.edu

H.-J. Senn and F. Otto (eds.), *Clinical Cancer Prevention*,
Recent Results in Cancer Research 188, DOI: 10.1007/978-3-642-10858-7_1,

1

posed the question of whether societal financial resources should be redirected to cancer prevention and early detection to us. In this chapter, we make select comments about how to be more selective in expenditures across the cancer care continuum. However, we fundamentally stress that in most societies, the choice of spending on prevention versus treatment is not an "either/or" option since the costs are noninterchangeable "societal silos." We also highlight our American perspective or limited vision of these topics.

1.2 Our Life Expectancy and Cancer Success Stories

The incidence and mortality rates for many cancers are modestly declining for the four most common cancers (Edwards et al. 2010). The relative contribution to primary prevention (e.g., smoking and lung cancer), early detection (mammography and colonoscopy), and improved treatment (principally adjuvant therapy) are hard to distinguish (Berry et al. 2005; Mandelblatt et al. 2009).

Primary prevention likely predominantly explains the gains in life expectancy in the prime years of life. A recent report noted that probability of deaths in the males in the prime years of life (ages 15–60) have declined by over 50% in Australia, Sweden, and the United States predominantly due to a decline in coronary artery disease and to a lesser extent cancer (Murray and Frenk 2010). In addition, the rates of death in Australia in young men are now about 40% lower than in the United States. Such a wide difference in premature deaths is more attributable to health behaviors (smoking, obesity, and physical inactivity) than treatments (hypertension, cancer) and early detection.

Despite, the modest declines in the four most common cancers in the United States, the relative frequency and mortality (except for the lymphomas) have changed little over the recent decades. Therefore, cancer now accounts for more deaths in individuals before age 85 than coronary artery disease (Jemal et al. 2009).

Current estimates indicate that about two-thirds of cancer burden as reflected in life years lost are preventable. Primary prevention is dominated by reducing tobacco use. The return of investment from reducing tobacco use and promoting smoking cessation is high – that is cost per unit of benefit that is low to approaching financial neutral when overall benefits from cancer, heart, and emphysema are aggregated.

Cancers associated with viral infections (hepatitis B and C, papilloma, and HIV) are a well-understood constellation of conditions. The relative burden of these infections as a cancer cause is inversely related to a countries relative affluence and sanitation infrastructure. The prevention benefits from selected vaccinations and sanitation (hepatitis C and *Helicobacter pylori*) have the greatest economic return since the cancer benefits are intertwined with other major health conditions (cirrhosis, diarrheal illness). Wisely in most affluent countries, beneficial cancer viral-associated vaccines are widely available if not optimally utilized.

1.3 No Cure in Sight: Costs of Drugs, Gadgets, Genomics and Technology

The United States spends 15–16% (more than $2 trillion) of its gross domestic product on health care. The United States spends 30–50% per capita before and after the adjustment of the relative income than European countries or Japan. What is more telling is that *all* these countries are experiencing an annual rate of growth of healthcare spending that is 2% per year, which is greater than their respective incomes from 1970 to 2006 (Aaron and Ginsburg 2009). In our opinion, the debate about the relative value of oncology innovations is most visible, vocal, and contentious in the United States in part due to the lack of meaningful restrains on pricing and diffusion into routine practice (after regulatory approval) (Bach 2009; Meropol and Schulman 2007). The collision between the need to control or slow the growth of expenditures and the moral imperative to save or prolong life is (finally) beginning to be publically discussed.

Cancer care costs account for only 5–10% of overall healthcare spending but this proportion is rapidly growing (Meropol et al. 2009). All countries are struggling with the financial burden associated with cancer and its treatment. In the United States, the most recent estimates from the National Cancer Institute from 2004 to 2006 are summarized in Table 1.1. In this 2-year period, overall expenditures were estimated to grow by 43%! The rates of growth for specific cancer types and the authors speculation on the predominant cause are listed below: lymphomas 117% – widespread use of rituximab; ovarian 95%, switch to docetaxel/carboplatin compared to generic paclitaxel; breast 72%, trastuzumab, dose-dense adjuvant therapy, plus more and different chemotherapy for metastatic disease; and kidney, the 2006 approval and use of sunitinib and sorafenib. The pressure to use the newest therapeutic and diagnostic technology in cancer treatment is intense and unrelenting force with only modest differs across the affluent countries of the world.

Worldwide, drugs associated with cancer care are estimated to cost ~$40 billion per year. In the United States, cancer drugs now represent the biggest category of overall pharmaceutical sales, growing at double the overall market; in

Table 1.1 Growth in US cancer expenditures

Cancer	% New cases	2004 Expenditures ($)	2006 Expenditures ($)	% Change
Lung	12.7	9.6	10.3	7.3
Breast	15.9	8.1	13.9	71.6
Colorectal	10.7	8.4	12.1	44.0
Prostate	16.8	8.0	9.7	21.3
Lymphoma	4.6	4.6	10.0	117.4
Head/neck	2.8	3.2	3.1	−3.1
Bladder	4.4	2.9	3.5	20.7
Leukemia	2.4	2.6	4.5	73.1
Ovary	1.9	2.2	4.3	95.5
Kidney	2.6	1.9	3.0	57.9
Endometrial	2.9	1.8	2.3	27.8
Cervix	0.8	1.7	1.4	−17.6
Pancreas	2.3	1.5	1.9	26.7
Melanoma	4.0	1.5	1.9	26.7
Esophagus	1.0	0.8	1.1	37.5
All other	14.0	13.4	20.6	53.7
Total	100	72.1	103.6	43.7

Author's modification of data abstracted from the National Cancer Institute's Cancer Trends Report (http:/progressreport.cancer.gov; accessed March 10, 2010)

1

2007 alone, sales increased by ~14%. Seventy percent of these sales come from products introduced in the last decade and 30% in the last 5 years (Gavel 2008). Currently, there are about 100 new molecules in phase III trials.

Additional evidence of the growing impact of cancer drug expenditures is from the annual projections for the US American Society of Health System Pharmacists that aggregate data from their member hospitals as well as national pharmacy benefit companies. Table 1.2 shows that antineoplastics are now the leading class in hospital drug expenditures (Hoffman et al. 2009). Table 1.3 rank orders expenditures for the 15 most expensive ambulatory drug classes of which 8 of 15 are for cancer. In 2005–2006, ambulatory drug expenditures grew by 20.8% and then declined in 2006–2007 to 9.9% associated predominantly with a marked decrease in erythropoiesis-stimulating agents used for kidney disease and cancer (Hoffman et al. 2008; 2009) Another recent projection over a longer time period of 1997–2004 and limited to Medicare expenditures only found that Part B drugs – a category dominated by cancer agents – grew from $3 billion to $11 billion (an increase of 267%) while the overall increase in Medicare spending increased 47% (Bach 2009). From 2005 to 2009, more than 90% of the anticancer agents approved by the FDA cost >$20,000 for a 12-week course of treatment (Fojo and Grady 2009).

While cancer drugs are the dominant drivers of the increasing cancer care costs, there are other factors. Technologic advances with high capital costs for equipment, e.g., the medical "arms race" is attributed to account for about one-half of recent overall health expenditure growth (Cutler 2006; Meropol et al. 2009) Specific cancer examples include the diffusion of positron emission tomography into general use, the selected use of robotics in surgery, and the increasing use of proton therapy instead of photons in radiation treatment (Mitchell 2008; Peeters in press; Hu et al. 2009).

In our opinion, the absolute financial impact of changes in cancer imaging and surgery are relatively modest since in most instances, practitioners are *switching* from one approach to another – e.g., using PET instead of CT scanning or robotic surgery instead of traditional approaches. In contrast, in medical oncology most evaluations of new molecules in clinical trials have investigated the *addition* of a new therapy – Drug A + B versus Drug A – making

Table 1.2 2007 US Hospital drug expenditures by class and change 2006–2007 (modified from Hoffman et al. 2009)

Drug class	Total 2007 ($ thousands)	% Total	2006–2007 (%)
Antineoplastics	3,321,432	12.2	6.6
Hemostatic modifiers	3,308,712	12.1	4.4
Anti-infectives, systemic	3,062,470	11.2	2.6
Blood growth factors	2,531,955	9.3	−11.2
Biologicals	1,552,058	6	22.2
Diagnostic aids	1,472,772	5	−1.3
Hospital solutions	1,468,450	5	23.8
Psychotherapeutics	1,134,477	4	1.3
Gastrointestinal	1,078,886	4	2.9
Respiratory therapy	984,172	4	9.9

Table 1.3 2008 US Ambulatory top 15 drug expenditures (modified from Hoffman et al. 2009)

Drug	2008 Expenditures ($ thousands)	% Change
Epoetin alfa (Procrit, Epogen)	2,668,665	–7.3
Pegfilgrastim (Neulasta)	1,690,977	4.6
Darbepoetin alfa (Aranesp)	1,158,329	–32.6
Infliximab (Remicade)	1,514,484	10.4
Bevacizumab (Avastin)	1,501,741	16.3
Rituximab (Rituxan)	1,347,430	11.4
Trastuzumab (Herceptin)	820,421	6.9
Oxaliplatin (Eloxatin)	809,380	5.1
Docetaxel (Taxotere)	666,224	14.3
Ranibizumab (Lucentis)	589,386	1.4
Varicella vaccine (Varivax)	569,569	19.1
HPV vaccine (Gardasil)	469,317	–5.5
Zoledronic acid (Zometa)	466,183	17.7
Gemcitabine (Gemzar)	425,591	8.2
Paricalcitol (Zemplar)	392,264	19.5

it impossible to confirm that standard therapy is still necessary (Dodwell et al. 2009).

1.4 Bending the Cancer Cost Curve

So what should cancer care providers do the "bend" the cancer care cost curve? The following is a chapter using the American television analogy of a ten best list. We believe that these steps can make a meaningful and long-term change in the trajectory of costs without compromising life expectancy and probably improving quality of life and end of life satisfaction (Table 1.4).

First, oncologists (as well as all physicians) must recognize that we drive the costs of care by what we do and don't do (Smith and Hillner in press). While American practitioners have more financial conflicts of interests than providers in other countries, almost all providers benefit from the use of more services (ownership in facilities, chemotherapy markups, name recognition, their reputations as centers of excellence, or simply covering their salary). What is less transparent is

Table 1.4 10 Steps to bending the cancer care cost curve

1. Acknowledge that we *drive* the costs of care by what we do, and don't do
2. Limit active therapy to patients with high performance status
3. Increase targeted therapy and use biologic imaging to limit ineffective therapies
4. Limit Nth-line therapy to patients previously responding or prolonged stable disease
5. For many cancer types, use sequential monotherapy for metastatic disease
6. Restrict red and white cell-stimulating factors to curative intent therapy
7. Provide tools to care providers to "reset" patient's unrealistic expectations of benefit
8. Reducing fears of abandonment with better less costly end of life care
9. Readjust compensation to rebalance cognitive services and disease-directed treatment
10. Accept the need for and guidance from cost-effectiveness analysis

that oncologists greatly influence patient's decision making in how care options are framed (Siminoff and Fetting 1989). Treatment benefits are predominantly expressed as relative not absolute benefits, prognosis, and anticipated survival are infrequently discussed or overly optimistic, and quality of life assumed to be maintained with treatment since something is being done without fully disclosing toxicity.

Active cancer-directed therapy should be limited to patients with high performance status and documented at each visit. While this requirement generally is not a major hurdle for adjuvant breast or colorectal patients, it would markedly reduce the frequency of therapy for many patients with lung cancer, the elderly in general, and patients considering second-line or late chemotherapy for metastatic disease. This is a classic concern of projecting the efficacy from clinical trials where usually >90% of patients have ECOG scores of 0 or 1 to the effectiveness of therapy in routine care.

Third, we are cautiously optimistic about expanding the use of genetic testing for selected cancer situations. While the evidence base needs to be strengthened by prospective validation, the key point is that the costs of these stratification tools will be offset by the treatment and toxicity costs avoided. A parallel approach is to use biologic imaging (currently predominantly PET-CT) to make earlier decisions during a course of therapy about stopping ineffective care.

Fourth, for cancer types where second, third, or more courses are potentially used, these should be explicitly limited to patients previously responding or having prolonged stable disease to the most immediate treatment. Giving second-line therapy to lung and breast cancer patients who had evidence of progression especially in the first 60 days of first-line therapy is wasteful, toxic, and detracts from the effective palliative care.

Fifth, for many cancers, sequential monotherapy offers less toxicity, improved quality of life, and no difference in overall survival. In addition, the need for supportive care drugs, their costs, and care visits are avoided. Combination therapies should be limited to curative intent and adjuvant therapy in most settings.

Sixth, restrict red and white cell growth factors to curative intent therapy. The use of erythropoiesis-stimulating agents has markedly declined due to safety concerns. Increasing concerns also apply to bisphosphonates. The long-standing debate about the need to maintain dose schedule or relative dose intensity is ongoing and skewed by pharmaceutical marketing. In our opinion, curative intent therapy (primarily adjuvant breast and lymphomas) is the only setting that can make a strong case for their use compared to dose reduction.

Seventh, "reset" patient's unrealistic expectations of benefit in making informed decisions by explicating outlining absolute benefits. While the majority of patients and their families use the Internet to boost their hopes of finding effective therapies, our impression is that it is only a minority that switches thorough numerous providers shopping for something better. We believe that much of the expectations are the result of their oncologist's failure to discuss advance directives before death is imminent. Our work among others have shown that patients want these conversations, they do not inflict emotional pain or depression, and there are clear benefits in more family communication, life planning, legacy/life review, and spiritual coping calmness. Better prognostic tools may be the catalyst for oncologist getting "real" sooner and recalibrate their common over optimism.

Eight, better less costly end of life care is possible especially when patient's fear of abandonment are explicitly addressed. Figure 1.1 shows a striking pattern in the United States, according to which, across most cancer types, 70–80% of the expenditure in the last year of the patient's life is mainly because of hospitalization (Yabroff et al. 2008). In addition, the average US Medicare, elderly beneficiary spends about 30% of his lifetime expenditures in that last year and 12–15% of it in the last month of life. While hospice use has been increased over time, the percent of patients who use hospice in the last 3 days of life is also increasing. More than 35% of overall hospice stays are 7 days or less (NHPCO 2010). As an extension of our prior points, we believe that fears of abandonment limit the use and earlier initiation of hospice. Again, framing the presentation from treating the cancer to controlling pain, dyspnea, constipation, etc. and focusing on assisting life transitions will lead to reduced costs and modulates expectations.

At least in the United States, there is a need to readjust compensation to rebalance cognitive services and disease-directed treatment. Some form of monthly management fees or illness-based payments is needed. Many oncologists practice with a sense of responsibility and availability that is 24/7/365. If we are going to change the financial incentives to save total cancer care costs, this must be done in a way that balances the professional lifestyle needs too.

We have had long careers making cost-effectiveness projections based on combining clinical trial efficacy with community reimbursement data. These projections have influenced some decisions in the United States, but the failure to have a central center for comparative effectiveness and to explicitly consider costs in the reimbursement approval decisions have made the impact of the field modest. We have long been convinced that doctors should not be rationing at the bedside (Iglehart 2009; Garber and Tunis 2009). An independent agency with the public interest and influence to healthcare budgets system widely appears finally to be coming to the United States as part of healthcare reform. While the National Institute of Clinical Effectiveness (NICE) is not perfect, it is a

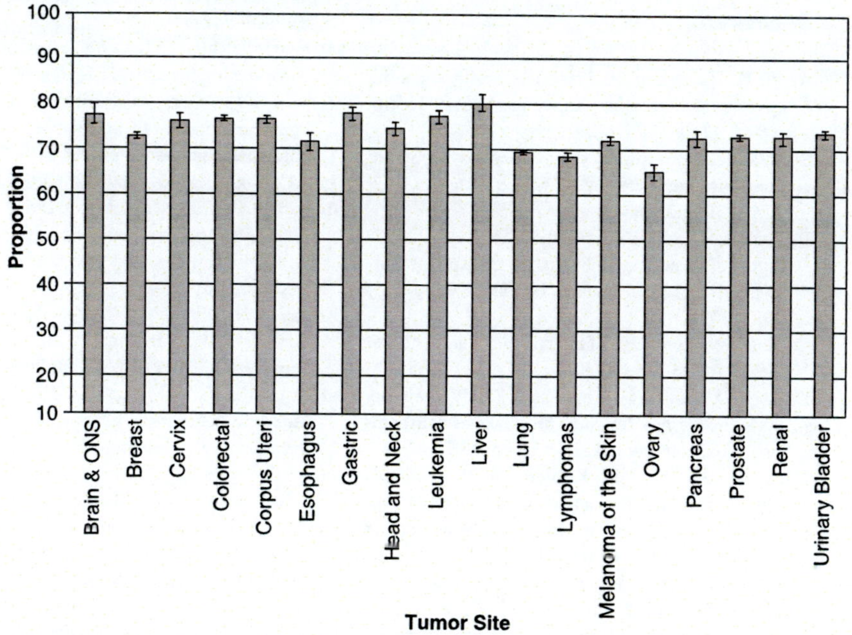

Fig. 1.1 Proportion of US net costs from hospitalizations in the last year of life phase (modified from Yabroff et al. 2008)

1

reasonable model for the *process* for the United States to emulate (Steinbrook 2008).

1.5 Conclusion

In most countries, the allocation of financial resources for cancer prevention, early detection, and treatment come from different nonrelated "silos." Primary prevention benefits have the greatest economic return since the cancer benefits are intertwined with other major health conditions. The costs of cancer care are rising faster any other area of the health care. Changing behaviors, incentives, expectations, and the framing of treatment effects are necessary to "bend" the current unrelenting cancer care cost curve.

References

Aaron HJ, Ginsburg PB (2009) Is health spending excessive? If so, what can we do about it? Health Aff 28:1260–1275

Bach PB (2009) Limits on Medicare's ability to control rising spending on cancer drugs. N Engl J Med 360:626–633

Berry DA, Cronin KA, Plevritis SK et al (2005) Effect of screening and adjuvant therapy on mortality from breast cancer. N Engl J Med 353: 1784–1792

Cutler DM Making sense of medical technology. (2006) Health Aff 25(2):w48–50

Dodwell D, Thorpe H, Coleman R (2009) Refining systemic therapy for early breast cancer: difficulties with subtraction. Lancet Oncol 10:738–739

Edwards BK, Ward E, Kohler BA et al (2010) Annual report to the nation on the status of cancer, 1975–2006, featuring colorectal cancer trends and impact of interventions (risk factors, screening, and treatment) to reduce future rates. Cancer 116:544–573

Fojo T, Grady C (2009) How much is life worth: cetuximab, non-small cell lung cancer, and the $440 billion question. J Natl Cancer Inst 101:1044–1048

Garber AM, Tunis SR (2009) Does comparative-effectiveness research threaten personalized medicine? N Engl J Med 360:1925–1927

Gavel S (2008) The oncology pipeline: maturing, competitive and growing. oncology business review 2008;September:14–17

Hoffman JM, Shah ND, Vermeulen LC et al (2008) Projecting future drug expenditures – 2008. Am J Health Syst Pharm 65:234–253

Hoffman JM, Shah ND, Vermeulen LC et al (2009) Projecting future drug expenditures – 2009. Am J Health Syst Pharm 66:237–257

Hu JC, Gu X, Lipsitz SR et al (2009) Comparative effectiveness of minimally invasive vs open radical prostatectomy. Jama 302:1557–1564

Iglehart JK (2009) Prioritizing comparative-effectiveness research – IOM recommendations. N Engl J Med 361:325–328

Jemal A, Siegel R, Ward E, Hao Y, Xu J, Thun MJ (2009) Cancer statistics, 2009. CA Cancer J Clin 59:225–49

Mandelblatt JS, Cronin KA, Bailey S et al (2009) Effects of mammography screening under different screening schedules: model estimates of potential benefits and harms. Ann Intern Med 151:738–747

Mcropol NJ, Schulman KA (2007) Cost of cancer care: issues and implications. J Clin Oncol 25:180–186

Meropol NJ, Schrag D, Smith TJ, et al. (2009) American Society of Clinical Oncology Guidance Statement: the cost of cancer care. J Clin Oncol JCO.2009.23.1183

Mitchell JM (2008) Utilization trends for advanced imaging procedures: evidence from individuals with private insurance coverage in California. Med Care 46:460–466

Murray CJL, Frenk J (2010) Ranking 37th – measuring the performance of the US Health Care System. N Engl J Med 362:98–99

NHPCO Facts and Figures: Hospice Care in America. National Hospice and Palliative Care Organization. less.http://www.nhpco.org/files/public/Statistics_Research/NHPCO_facts_and_figures.pdfAccessed March 12, 2010

Peeters A, Grutters JPC, Pijls-Johannesma M et al (2010) How costly is particle therapy? Cost analysis of external beam radiotherapy with carbon-ions, protons and photons. Radiother Oncol. 2010 Apr;95(1):45–53. Epub 2010 Jan 26

Siminoff LA, Fetting JH (1989) Effects of outcome framing on treatment decisions in the real

world: Impact of framing on adjuvant breast cancer decisions. Med Dec Making 9(4):262–271
Smith T, Hillner B (2010) Concrete options and ideas for increasing value in oncology care: the view from one trench. Oncologist. 2010;15 Suppl 1:65–72
Steinbrook R (2008) Saying no isn't NICE – the travails of Britain's National Institute for Health and Clinical Excellence. N Engl J Med 359: 1977–1981
Yabroff KR, Lamont EB, Mariotto A et al (2008) Cost of care for elderly cancer patients in the United States. J Natl Cancer Inst 100:630–641

Lessons Learned from Prevention Programs: Different Endpoints Should Be Used in Secondary and Tertiary Prevention

2

Franz Porzsolt

Abstract It is mandatory to compare cost and consequences of healthcare services if public support is requested. This request will apply to all healthcare services including prevention. As the demand for health care will always exceed the available resources, methods that make it possible to select the "best" programs for implementation have to be developed. The selection of the "best" programs is not easy because there exist so far no generally accepted quality criteria that can be used to identify the "best" prevention programs.

Based on a model on structural and functional properties of a disease, it is concluded that the traditional outcomes of treatment and prevention may be useful for the evaluation of tertiary prevention programs, but not of secondary prevention programs. Neither the traditional endpoints of treatment studies nor traditional surrogate parameters are useful for the evaluation of secondary prevention programs.

Using the assumptions of the model and a list of available data in secondary prevention programs we recommend to assess five indicators for description of the value of a secondary prevention program: quality of life, surrogates for life expectancy, the perspective of the assessor, the conditions of assessment, and finally the payment. As each of these five items offers two possible values prevention programs may be classified into 32 different groups.

2.1 Introduction

It has long been recognized that economic analyses of prevention programs should be completed (Broudy et al. 1979; Dalziel and Segal 2006; Foster et al. 2003; Holtgrave et al. 1996; Manau et al. 1987; Tager and Sondik 1985; Wang et al. 2006). The special problem of most prevention programs is the long time period between their intervention and outcome. This is probably the reason that most economic evaluations are confined to the description of costs (Foster et al. 2003; Manau et al. 1987), discuss the interventions that are necessary to reduce the risk of disease (Holtgrave et al. 1996 Mahoney et al), or discuss the uncertainty of the economic analysis of prevention programs (Dalziel and Segal 2006; Wang et al. 2006).

The structure and the process of most prevention programs are described in detail but

F. Porzsolt
Clinical Economics, University of Ulm,
Frauensteige 6, 89075, Ulm, Germany
e-mail: franz.porzsolt@uniklinik-ulm.de

H.-J. Senn and F. Otto (eds.), *Clinical Cancer Prevention*,
Recent Results in Cancer Research 188, DOI: 10.1007/978-3-642-10858-7_2,

almost no information is available on the achievement of the finally intended outcomes. The expected outcomes are usually well defined and there are several surrogate parameters, which refer to promising results. The validity of these intermediate results depends on the mode of assessment (under experimental or under day-to-day) conditions. The results may be assessed by healthcare providers or healthcare users. Depending on the assessed topic and on the conditions of assessments, the meaning of the assessed outcome and the value of the prevention program may be quite different. The economic decisions may include several aspects such as financial resources, research manpower, the chance to succeed, and the reduction of ineffective programs applied to our patients.

We shall not be satisfied with preliminary data and with the fact that most prevention programs are dangling their final results. We should provide data which describe the information and the interventions are offered to the healthcare users, i.e., people at risk. We have to record the behavior of this group of people, i.e., the adherence to our recommendations and to document different types of comprehensible outcomes.

This paper describes a Gedanken experiment (Mach 1976; Popper 1968) that generated an algorithm, which can be used to evaluate various prevention programs according to the patients' perspective.

2.2 Methods

The Gedanken experiment is based on three assumptions.

- First, a disease can be detected by structural and/or functional properties. The structures can be described by macroscopic, microscopic, or biomolecular features, i.e., laboratory tests or imaging methods. The functions of a disease can be detected by the effects of a disease on a persons' quality of life or life expectancy.
- Second, functional properties of a disease are more important than structural properties. Examples are shown in Table 2.1. These examples demonstrate that functional properties of a disease are more important than structural properties: prostate cancer is frequently detected by structural properties, which are detected by digital rectal examination. Many of the detected prostate cancer affect neither the quality of life nor the life expectancy. In patients with cancer of unknown primary the absence of detectable structures does not rule out the disease but may have considerable effects on both quality and quantity of life.
- Third, diagnostic systems, which focus structural but no functional properties of diseases – like many of our staging systems – cannot be used for the assessment of secondary prevention programs.

Table 2.1 Structural and functional properties of diseases. Structural properties are described by anatomical features (macroscopic, microscopic, and biomolecular). Functional properties of diseases influence the physiology of a person such as the quality of life or the life expectancy. Examples are derived from malignant diseases

		Functional properties of diseases	
		Frequently detected	Rarely detected
Structural properties of diseases	Frequently detected	Most forms of cancer	Prostate cancer
	Rarely detected	Cancer of primary unknown	Death of unknown reason

These three assumptions provide the basis for the categorization of traditional outcomes. As these traditional outcomes are not really useful for the assessment of the value of secondary prevention programs we propose different criteria for secondary and tertiary prevention. These criteria have to be measurable, available, and interpretable.

2.3 Results

2.3.1 Traditional Outcomes of Treatment and of Prevention Programs

Prevention programs in this paper are structured according to the different phases in the natural history of a disease as described by Baselga and Senn (2008). The expected goals of these programs are the prevention of either the appearance of a disease (i.e., primary prevention). This aspect of prevention is *not* included in our analysis. Other important goals are the prevention of disease progression (i.e., secondary prevention including screening) or the prevention of the fatal consequences of a disease (i.e., tertiary prevention). When these final goals are critically analyzed six theoretical outcomes can be described (Fig. 2.1).

One of the most frequently observed final outcome of a prevention program is nonadherence due to other priorities. Although nonadherence is rarely quantified it is well known and several strategies were recommended to overcome this problem (Bosch-Capblanch et al. 2007; DeKosky 2006; DiMatteo 2003; Ebrahim 1998; Hiatt 1997; Rockson 2009; Stirratt and Gordon 2008).

The explicitly intended outcome of secondary prevention is cure. It is definitely not difficult to identify the failures of secondary prevention as these patients undergo palliative therapy and will either be able to survive with cancer or have to continue palliative therapy as long as its benefit outbalances its harm. Patients who survive with cancer belong to the group in Table 2.1 in which structures but no functions of the disease are detectable. Patients who need palliative therapy will finally succumb to functions of the disease either without or with detectable structures of the disease.

The identification of patients who will be cured even without prevention is more difficult because nearly all patients with a confirmed positive screening result will undergo treatment. These patients who are cured either with or without treatment belong to the group in Table 2.1 in which neither structures nor functions of the disease are detectable. Except from very few special situations there will be no population in which the "natural course" of the disease can be investigated. Such a "special situation" emerged when mass screening of women for breast cancer was introduced in Norway. Zahl et al. (2008) used a rather intelligent approach to identify the number of breast cancer cases that were detected with and without mammography. As there is positive evidence, which seems to exclude several possibilities to explain this observation (Kaplan and Porzsolt 2008), the most likely explanation favors the interpretation that about 20% of invasive breast cancers that are detected by screening mammography will regress spontaneously (Porzsolt and Hölzel 2009).

In addition to the final outcomes a large series of surrogate parameters is assessed following secondary prevention programs. The assessed surrogates are related to the investigated interventions or are obtained from special tests. Examples of interventions are lifestyle changes or treatments. Suggested lifestyle changes were exercise, weight management, healthy diet, moderate alcohol consumption, and fruit and vegetable intake (Cummings et al. 2009). The recommended treatments include oophorectomy (Metcalfe 2009), treatment with

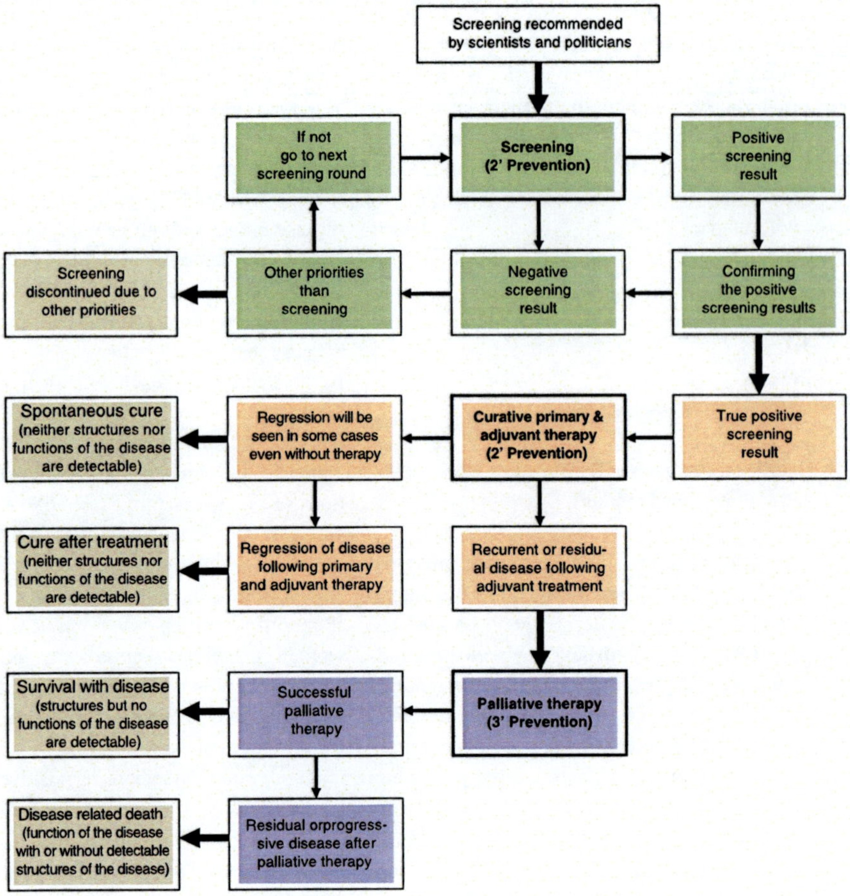

Fig. 2.1 Theoretical outcomes following secondary and tertiary prevention. For complete evaluation all persons who were included in a screening program have to be considered. A complete evaluation has to differentiate among six different outcomes: discontinuation of screening, survival with disease, survival without disease due to effective treatment or due to spontaneous cure, death due to the screened disease, and finally – not shown here – death of unknown reason

phytochemicals (Adams and Chen 2009), selective estrogen receptor modulators (Li and Brown 2009; Howell et al. 2008; Powles 2008; Wickerham et al. 2009), retionoids (Bonanni and Lazzeroni 2009), bisphosphonates (Valachis et al. 2010), nonsteroidal anti-inflammatory drugs (Agrawal and Fentiman 2008), or vitamin D (Welsh 2007).

In other studies it is claimed that the risk of breast cancer can be predicted, e.g., by intraductal tests such as nipple aspiration fluid, ductal lavage, mammary ductoscopy, or periareolar fine needle aspiration (Cazzaniga et al. 2009)

In summary, the traditional endpoints of treatment may be useful in tertiary prevention programs but are not helpful for secondary prevention when the success following screening and the subsequent treatment has to be described. None of the assessed surrogate parameters could reliably predict the success of secondary prevention. Therefore, it is necessary to search for new indicators of successful secondary prevention programs.

2.3.2 Proposal for the Evaluation of Prevention Programs

The traditional endpoints of treatment studies such as cure or survival will only rarely be reported following secondary and tertiary prevention and are therefore considered as theoretical outcomes of prevention programs. From a scientific point of view, it is often not possible to differentiate between spontaneous cure, treatment-related cure, or survival with disease. Therefore, the traditional endpoints are no ideal candidates when measurable endpoints are needed for comparative evaluations especially of secondary prevention programs.

On the other hand there is sufficient information in most secondary and tertiary prevention programs on aspects such as practicability, demand, compliance, and side effects. These criteria are correlated with the final endpoints of secondary and tertiary prevention programs because they all influence the adherence to the program and are signs of program success or failure.

Prevention is usually demanded by patients because it induces hope and confidence. The demand will be correlated at least with short-term adherence, and this can be quantified. In some programs adherence was quantified and may even predict survival (Bauer et al. 2010; Martín-López and Hernández-Barrera 2010), a result which has to be interpreted with care.

The effects of prevention are sometimes assessed under day-to-day conditions and sometimes only under the experimental conditions of a study. Even this information on the condition can be used as indicator for the value of a prevention program.

It can also be assessed if the effects of a program are self-assessed by the patients or are assessed by proxy raters and finally the payer of a prevention program, private or public, can be identified.

This information can be used for the evaluation of prevention programs because it is frequently available, easy to record, and describes at least some aspects of the value of prevention programs.

Considering this information, which is available in most prevention programs, and the lessons that were derived from the three above assumptions, five levels of outcomes that consider

Table 2.2 Efficiency of secondary prevention programs. One of two possible answers has to be selected at each of five levels (A–E). The chosen order among and within the levels A–E is justified in the text. The higher the resulting five digit number, the higher is the efficiency of the prevention program (e.g., 11101 is considered more efficient than 11011)

Level	(A)	(B)	(C)	(D)	(E)
Direct (1) or no direct (0) effect on quality of life	(1/0)				
Effect (1) or no effect (0) on surrogate of life expectancy		(1/0)			
Prioritized effect assessed under day-to-day conditions (1) or under experimental (0) conditions			(1/0)		
Prioritized effect is self-assessed (1) or proxy rated (0)				(1/0)	
Prevention is financed by private (1) or public (0) resources					(1/0)

functional aspects of disease management are proposed (Table 2.2). These aspects are quality of life (A), life expectancy (B), the perspective of the assessor (C), the conditions of assessment (D), and finally the payment (E).

Quality of life (A) refers not only to aspects that are recorded by quality of life instruments but also to any behavior that can be explained as action to optimize the quality of life (Magai et al. 2007). An example for differences in optimizing the quality of life may be the two groups of women who accept or do not accept mammography. Although we cannot be sure that the sender and the receiver of information will perceive the same message at least one of the two target populations, i.e., women who accept mammography, obviously consider the benefit of mammography higher than the psychological stress and discomfort associated with mammography while women who refuse mammography interpret the identical information differently. The acceptance rate of a prevention program may therefore be a useful indicator for the effect of a prevention program on the quality of life. Well-accepted prevention programs are expected to have a more favorable effect on the quality of life than rarely accepted programs.

The possibility to influence the own life expectancy (B) is always an important aspect for decision making. The strong request of screening supports the assumption that patients wish to contribute to improve their life expectancy. As we have begun to understand the factors that influence these decisions (Misono et al. 2008), the number of appropriate surrogate parameters, which indicate positive effects on the patients' life expectation, will increase. Therefore, the indicators of life expectancy were included in the list of criteria for evaluation of prevention programs.

The perspective of the person who makes the assessment (C) has a considerable influence on the described outcome. Quality of life assessment is an example for the huge differences that can be observed when quality of life is self-assessed or assessed by a proxy rater. Self-assessments are higher rated than proxy ratings also in the evaluation of prevention programs.

The important influence of assessment conditions (D) are not always considered carefully enough. In the scientific literature efficacy and effectiveness are differentiated. Efficacious programs are assessed by *healthcare providers* under *ideal but artificial* conditions. Effective programs are assessed by *healthcare providers* under *day-to-day* conditions. Although these definitions are used by some groups (Ernst and Canter 2005; Porzsolt et al. 2010) they are not commonly accepted. Effects that are observed under day-to-day conditions are considered more important than effects observed under ideal but artificial conditions.

Finally, we consider the payer (E) of the prevention program. Prevention programs that require public resources are considered less valuable than programs that are privately financed.

Among the five criteria for assessment of the value the measurable effects on quality of life were estimated higher than surrogate parameters for the life expectancy. The effects on these two outcomes were followed by the condition under which the data were generated and recorded because this information will be more often contributed to the evaluation than the information on the rater of the effect. In addition to the information on the rater the information on the payer was considered the least important aspect for description of the value of a prevention program.

2.4 Discussion

2.4.1 The Risk of Interpretation in Prevention Programs

It is not easy to interpret data from prevention programs as the true reasons of the observed effects may be generally expected. So it is commonly

assumed that strong adherence to guidelines or to recommendations of prevention programs will result in extension of life expectancy. There are even grants, which are provided for projects to demonstrate a correlation of adherence to recommendations and increased life expectancy.
The correct interpretation may be quite complicated as it should be excluded that patients with less complications and a less problematic course of the disease will be those who can follow the recommendations more closely than patients with complications or side effects of incompatibilities. In other words, especially in secondary prevention programs there are several possible confounders, which have to be excluded to avoid misinterpretation of the obtained data.

The value of prevention programs from the patients' perspectives is not identical to the perspectives of other stakeholders. Patients as well as persons at risks of health problems are satisfied if a prevention program restores the lost health or prevents the loss of health. Other stakeholders such as doctors, hospital managers, health insurance companies, or politicians strive for additional goals. None of these partners will be satisfied if only the patients' goals will be achieved by prevention. The endeavor to reach additional goals is absolutely justified. The emerging risk is associated with a potential imbalance between the patients' goals and the goals of any other stakeholder. This risk can be avoided if we make sure that the patients' goals will be the primary goals of any healthcare prevention program and that at least part of the patients' goals are achieved to justify the expenditures for prevention. The described proposal describes a strategy for the assessment of the patients' value of prevention programs.

2.4.2 The Resulting Need for Evaluation of Preventive Medicine

The increasing demand for healthcare resources is justified by progress and innovations in health care. This progress and innovations have to be financed. Unless additional value is generated these investments inherit the risk of an economic hazard. The critical question therefore is what should be accepted as "added value" and for whom. These criteria will be different for treatments and tests. It is probably not justified to qualify a test as "added value," which just identifies a new target population without providing any further evidence, e.g., on the risk reduction that can be achieved in this newly identified population. A corresponding problem applies to any new preventive treatment, which generates promising surrogate parameters but no additional information on the final success of the prevention program. Our recently published strategy (Porzsolt et al. 2009) proposes a classification of innovations. This classification is based on the amount of available qualitative information. The more information is available, which quantifies the "added value," the higher is the recommendation for the public support of the investigated prevention program.

The strategy was developed to provide a solution for the general problem of healthcare prevention programs. This general problem emerges because our societies consider health care a public good without having commonly accepted indicators to evaluate the quality of this good.

For evaluating the quality of prevention programs the benefits and risks of prevention programs have to be defined. We have summarized a wide spectrum of different preventive treatments and a huge variety of surrogate parameters, which are applied to justify further research. These surrogate parameters are specific for the used treatment and are, therefore, difficult to compare. Two aspects should be considered in a scientifically sound analysis. First, the specificity of the applied treatment is more important than the specificity of the surrogate parameter. Second, the surrogate parameter but not the treatment has to be correlated with the intended final outcome. In other words, surrogate parameters cannot be used to confirm the specificity of

2

a prevention program but may be used to demonstrate the effectiveness of the program if the correlation of the surrogate with the final endpoint has been confirmed.

2.4.3 Recommendations for Future Preventive Research

It should be considered that the public demand for prevention programs is rather strong but the reasons of this strong demand are not well understood. It may be that screening programs for fatal diseases generate perceived safety, which can be quantified (Ursula Rochau, Thesis Medical Faculty University of Ulm 2009, Larissa Gampert, Thesis Medical Faculty University of Ulm 2010, Andreas Knie, Thesis Medical Faculty University of Ulm 2010) and is probably one of the most important aspects of quality of life. So far, most preventive research has been addressing only traditional endpoints, which are rarely achieved, or surrogates of these endpoints, which are not reliable indicators of the quality of a prevention program.

The distinction of structural and functional properties of a disease may be a helpful concept to accept additional markers for description of the quality of prevention programs. It is important in the future to identify functionally inert diseases such as most prostatic cancers, which can be diagnosed due to structural markers but do not need preventive treatment as these forms of cancer cause no harmful functions. This differentiated concept has been discussed in several research areas such as ophthalmology (Brown 2008), nutrition (Paukov 2007), pulmonary disease (Wedzicha and Hurst 2007), and in basic biomolecular research (Malavaki et al. 2008).

The specificity of a prevention program is another problem, which is barely discussed. Although this problem is one of the most complicated research problems and requires ambitious research strategies it should urgently be addressed. It may even be worth the establishment of a special task force. The related problem of "nondisease" is known for almost 50 years (Meador 1965) and has been supported by more recent work on the existence of nondisease genes (Osada et al. 2009). For those who are following these more basic considerations, it is not surprising that the US Prevention Services Task Force (USPSTF) revised their recommendations (regular breast cancer screening only at the age of 50, screening only every other year, neither encouraging nor teaching breast self-examination and no mammography beyond 75). The new findings and the recommendations of a task force should be sufficient to trigger a discussion, which is directly related to the effectiveness and efficiency of today's medicine.

If preventive medicine wants to keep up with the progress in other areas of medicine it will be mandatory to establish standard rules for basic preventive research. These rules may include the description of the risk profiles of the target population, the investigated interventions, as well as the reported outcomes, which are discussed in this chapter. The resulting structure, which offers the distinction of 32 different values for secondary prevention programs, may serve as proposal for further discussions.

References

USPSTF. http://www.breastcancer.org/symptoms/testing/new_research

Adams LS, Chen S (2009) Phytochemicals for breast cancer prevention by targeting aromatase. Front Biosci 14:3846–3863

Agrawal A, Fentiman IS (2008) NSAIDs and breast cancer: a possible prevention and treatment strategy. Int J Clin Pract 62:444–449

Baselga J, Senn H-J (2008) The perspective and role of the medical oncologist in cancer prevention: a position paper by the European Society for Medical Oncology (editorial). Ann Oncol 19: 1033–1035. doi:10.1093/annonc/mdn366

Bauer T, Gitt AK, Jünger C, Zahn R, Koeth O, Towae F, Schwarz AK, Bestehorn K, Senges J, Zeymer U; for the Acute Coronary Syndromes Registry (ACOS) investigators (2010 Mar 25). Guideline-recommended secondary prevention drug therapy after acute myocardial infarction: predictors and outcomes of nonadherence. Eur J Cardiovasc Prev Rehabil [Epub ahead of print]

Bonanni B, Lazzeroni M (2009) Retinoids and breast cancer prevention. Recent Results Cancer Res 181:77–82

Bosch-Capblanch X, Abba K, Prictor M, Garner P (2007) Contracts between patients and healthcare practitioners for improving patients' adherence to treatment, prevention and health promotion activities. Cochrane Database Syst Rev (2), CD004808

Broudy DW, Swint JM, Lairson DR (1979) Prospective economic evaluation of lead poisoning prevention programs. J Community Health 4:291–301

Brown B (2008 Nov) Structural and functional imaging of the retina: new ways to diagnose and assess retinal disease. Clin Exp Optom 91(6): 504–14

Cazzaniga M, Decensi A, Bonanni B, Luini A, Gentilini O (2009) Biomarkers for risk assessment and prevention of breast cancer. Curr Cancer Drug Targets 9:482–499

Cummings SR, Tice JA, Bauer S, Browner WS, Cuzick J, Ziv E, Vogel V, Shepherd J, Vachon C, Smith-Bindman R, Kerlikowske K (2009) Prevention of breast cancer in postmenopausal women: approaches to estimating and reducing risk. J Natl Cancer Inst 101:384–398

Dalziel K, Segal L (2006) Point: uncertainty in the economic analysis of school-based obesity prevention programs: urgent need for quality evaluation. Obesity 14:1481–1482

DeKosky ST (2006) Maintaining adherence and retention in dementia prevention trials. Neurology 67(Suppl 3):S14–16

DiMatteo MR (2003) Future directions in research on consumer-provider communication and adherence to cancer prevention and treatment. Patient Educ Couns 50:23–26

Ebrahim S (1998) Detection, adherence and control of hypertension for the prevention of stroke: a systematic review. Health Technol Assess 2:1–78

Ernst E, Canter PH (2005) Limitations of "pragmatic" trials. Postgrad Med J 81:203

Foster EM, Dodge KA, Jones D (2003) Issues in the economic evaluation of prevention programs. Appl Dev Sci 7:76–86

Ghosh PF, AK KRM (2009) Qualitative assessment of innovations in healthcare provision. BMC Health Serv Res 9:50

Hiatt RA (1997) Behavioral research contributions and needs in cancer prevention and control: adherence to cancer screening advice. Prev Med 26:S11–18

Holtgrave DR, Qualls NL, Graham JD (1996) Economic evaluation of HIV prevention programs. Annu Rev Public Health 17:467–488

Howell A, Bundred NJ, Cuzick J, Allred DC, Clarke R (2008) Response and resistance to the endocrine prevention of breast cancer. Adv Exp Med Biol 617:201–211

Kaplan RM, Porzsolt F (2008) The natural history of breast cancer. Arch Int Med 168:2302–2303

Li Y, Brown PH (2009) Prevention of ER-negative breast cancer. Recent Results Cancer Res 181: 121–134

Mach E (1976) On thought explanatory experiments. In: Mach E (ed) Knowledge and error: sketches on the psychology of enquiry. Reidel, Dordrecht (Translation of Erkenntnis und Irrtum, 5th edn, 1926).

Magai C, Consedine N, Neugut AI, Hershman DL (2007) Common psychosocial factors underlying breast cancer screening and breast cancer treatment adherence: a conceptual review and synthesis. J Womens Health 16:11–23

Mahoney MC, Bevers T, Linos E, Willett WC (2008) Opportunities and strategies for breast cancer prevention through risk reduction. CA Cancer J Clin 58:347–371

Malavaki C, Mizumoto S, Karamanos N, Sugahara K (2008) Recent advances in the structural study of functional chondroitin sulfate and dermatan sulfate in health and disease. Connect Tissue Res 49:133–139

Manau C, Cuenca E, Martínez-Carretero J, Salleras L (1987) Economic evaluation of community programs for the prevention of dental caries in Catalonia, Spain. Commun Dent Oral Epidemiol 15:297–300

Martín-López R, Hernández-Barrera V, Lopez De Andres A, Garrido PC, Gil De Miguel A, García RJ (2010) Breast and cervical cancer screening in Spain and predictors of adherence. Eur J Cancer Prev 19:227–238

2

Meador CK (1965) The art and science of nondisease. N Engl J Med 272:92–95

Metcalfe KA (2009) Oophorectomy for breast cancer prevention in women with BRCA1 or BRCA2 mutations. Womens Health 5:63–68

Misono S, Weiss NS, Fann JR, Redman M, Yueh B (2008) Incidence of suicide in persons with cancer. J Clin Oncol 26:4731–4738

Osada N, Mano S, Gojobori J (2009) Quantifying dominance and deleterious effect on human disease genes. Proc Natl Acad Sci USA 106: 841–846

Paukov VS (2007) Structural and functional conception of alcohol disease. Zh Nevrol Psikhiatr Im S S Korsakova Suppl 1:8–11

Popper K (1968) On the use and misuse of imaginary explanatory experiments, especially in quantum theory. In: Popper K (ed) The logic of scientific discovery. Harper Torch Books, New York, pp 442–456

Porzsolt F, Hölzel D (2009) Spontaneous remissions in breast cancer underline the need of more evidence: screening should not detect more cancer but earlier cancer. J Publ Health 18:15–19. doi:10.1007/s10389-009-0275-4

Porzsolt F, Eisemann M, Habs M (2010) Complementary alternative medicine and traditional scientific medicine should use identical rules to complete clinical trials. EUJIM 2:3–7. doi:10.1016/j.eujim.2010.02.001 http://dx.doi.org/10.1016/j.eujim.2010.02.001

Powles TJ (2008) Prevention of breast cancer using SERMs. Adv Exp Med Biol 630:232–236

Rockson SG (2009) Appropriate secondary prevention of acute atherothrombotic events and strategies to improve guideline adherence. Postgrad Med 121:25–39

Stirratt MJ, Gordon CM (2008) Adherence to biomedical HIV prevention methods: considerations drawn from HIV treatment adherence research. Curr HIV/AIDS Rep 5:186–192

Tager AM, Sondik EJ (1985) Economic evaluation of the benefits of cancer prevention and health promotion programs. Md Med J 34:77–82

Valachis A, Polyzos NP, Georgoulias V, Mavroudis D, Mauri D (2010) Lack of evidence for fracture prevention in early breast cancer bisphosphonate trials: a meta-analysis. Gynecol Oncol 117:139–145

Wang LY, Yang Q, Lowry R, Wechsler H (2006) Counterpoint: uncertainty in the economic analysis of school-based obesity prevention programs: urgent need for quality evaluation. Obesity 14:1483–1484

Wedzicha JA, Hurst JR (2007) Structural and functional co-conspirators in chronic obstructive pulmonary disease exacerbations. Proc Am Thorac Soc 4:602–605

Welsh J (2007) Vitamin D and prevention of breast cancer. Acta Pharmacol Sin 28:1373–1382

Wickerham DL, Costantino JP, Vogel VG, Cronin WM, Cecchini RS, Ford LG, Wolmark N (2009) The use of tamoxifen and raloxifene for the prevention of breast cancer. Recent Results Cancer Res 181:113–119

Zahl PH, Mæhlen J, Welch HG (2008) The natural course of invasive breast cancer detected by mammography. Arch Intern Med 168:2311–2316

Biomarkers for Early Detection and as Surrogate Endpoints in Cancer Prevention Trials: Issues and Opportunities

3

Barbara K. Dunn, Karin Jegalian, and Peter Greenwald

Abstract In order to improve the early detection and diagnosis of cancer, give more accurate prognoses, stratify individuals by risk, predict response to treatment, and help the transition of basic research into clinical application, biomarkers are needed that accurately represent or predict clinical outcomes. To be useful in trials for chemopreventive agent development, biomarkers must be subject to modulation, easy to obtain and quantify, and have biological meaning, ideally representing steps in well-understood carcinogenic pathways. Though difficult to validate fully, wisely chosen biomarkers in early-phase trials can inform the prioritization of large-scale, long-term trials that measure clinical outcomes. When well-designed, smaller trials using biomarkers as surrogate endpoints should promote faster decisions regarding which targeted preventive agents to pursue, promising greater progress in the personalization of medicine. Biomarkers could become useful in distinguishing indolent from aggressive forms of ductal carcinoma in situ as well as localized invasive breast and prostate cancer, lesions that are often overtreated. Chemopreventive strategies that reduce the progression of early forms of premalignancy can benefit patients not only by reducing their risk of cancer and death from cancer but also by reducing their need for invasive interventions. Genomic and proteomic methods offer the possibility of revealing new potential markers, especially for diseases whose biology is complex or not well understood. Panels of markers may be used to accommodate the molecular heterogeneity of cancers. Biomarkers in phase 2 prevention trials of combinations of chemopreventive drugs have been used to demonstrate synergistic action of multiple agents, allowing use of lower doses, with less toxicity, a critical feature of interventions intended for cancer prevention.

B.K. Dunn (✉) and P. Greenwald
Basic Prevention Science Research Group,
Division of Cancer Prevention, National Cancer Institute, 6130 Executive Boulevard, Room 2036, Bethesda, MD 20892-7340, USA
e-mail: dunnb@mail.nih.gov;
e-mail: greenwap@mail.nih.gov

K. Jegalian
Garrett Park, Bethesda, MD, USA
e-mail: karinjeg@verizon.net

Abbreviations

AI	Aromatase Inhibitor
ACS	American Cancer Society
APC	Adenoma Prevention with Celecoxib Trial
APC	Adenomatous polyposis coli gene
BCPT	Breast Cancer Prevention Trial

H.-J. Senn and F. Otto (eds.), *Clinical Cancer Prevention*,
Recent Results in Cancer Research 188, DOI: 10.1007/978-3-642-10858-7_3,

Bcl-2	B cell lymphoma 2 protein
BRCA	Breast cancer gene
CD10	A zinc-dependent metalloprotease enzyme
CDH1	Cadherin gene
CEA	Carcinoembryonic antigen
COX2	Cyclooxygenase 2
CT	Computed tomography
DCIS	Ductal carcinoma in situ
DCC	Deleted in Colorectal Cancer gene
DFMO	α-difluoromethylornithine
DHT	Dihydrotestosterone
DNA	Deoxyribonucleic acid
EDRN	Early Detection Research Network
EGF	Epidermal growth factor
EGFR	Epidermal growth factor receptor
ETS	E-twenty six
ETV	ETS translocation variant
ERG	ETS related gene
ER-	Estrogen receptor-negative
ER+	Estrogen receptor-positive
FDA	Food and Drug Administration
FHIT	Fragile Histidine Triad gene
GI	Gastrointestinal
GGO	Ground-glass opacity
HbA1C	Glycated hemoglobin
HER2	Human epidermal growth factor receptor 2
HPV	Human papilllomavirus
HRT	Hormone replacement therapy
IBC	Invasive breast cancer
IBIS	International Breast Intervention Study
IEN	Intra-epithelial neoplasia
IGF-1	Insulin-like growth factor 1
IGFBP-3	Insulin-like growth factor binding protein 3
Ki-67	A protein that in humans is encoded by the *MKI67* gene
KRAS	Kirsten ras sarcoma viral oncogene
LAMR1	laminin receptor 1
LGD1069	Bexarotene (Targretin)
MCM2	Minichromosome maintenance protein
MGMT	O6-methylguanine–DNA methyltransferase gene
MiB2	Breast cancer marker of proliferation
NCI	National Cancer Institute
NLST	National Lung Screening Trial
NSABP	National Surgical Adjuvant Breast and Bowel Project
NSAID	Non-steroidal anti-inflammatory drug
P53	A tumor suppressor protein that in humans is encoded by the *TP53* gene
P16	A tumor suppressor gene, also known as cyclin-dependent kinase inhibitor 2A (*CDKN2A*) gene
PARP	Poly (ADP-ribose) polymerase
PCNA	Proliferating cell nuclear antigen
PCA3	Prostate cancer antigen 3
PCPT	Prostate Cancer Prevention Trial
PCR	Polymerase chain reaction
PGP9.5	Protein gene product 9.5 gene
PLCO	Prostate, Lung, Colorectal and Ovarian Cancer Screening Trial
PR	Progesterone receptor
PSA	Prostate-specific antigen
PSMA	Prostate-specific membrane antigen
RASSF1A	Ras ASSociation domain Family 1A gene
RNA	Ribonucleic acid
RPFNA	Random periareolar fine-needle aspiration
RXR	Retinoid X receptor
S100A7	Protein S100-A7 encoded by the *S100A7* gene
SEB	Surrogate Endpoint Biomarker
SELECT	Selenium and Vitamin E Cancer Prevention Trial
SERMS	Selective estrogen receptor modulators
SPINK1	Pancreatic secretory trypsin inhibitor
STAR	Study of Tamoxifen and Raloxifene
SWOG	Southwest Oncology Group
TGFβ	Transforming growth factor beta
TMPRSS2	Transmembrane protease, serine 2

3.1 Biomarkers: What They Are and How They Are Applied

Biomarkers are physical entities or images of these entities that can be measured and used to indicate a biological process, disease process, or drug response (Wagner 2002). Examples of biomarkers that have become widely used in the clinic or in research settings include PSA (prostate specific antigen) to assess prostate cancer burden, Ki-67 as a marker for cell proliferation and therefore cancer, and C-reactive protein as a marker of inflammation. In noncancer settings, well-known biomarkers include blood pressure and serum lipids as measures for cardiovascular disease, hemoglobin A1C as a measure for blood sugar control in diabetes, and seropositivity to assess vaccine protection.

In cancer medicine biomarkers have been used for several purposes: to establish individual risk of disease; for classification and prediction, which includes screening markers for early detection, diagnostic markers in individuals with signs or symptoms, and "prognostic markers" that predict subsequent outcomes in patients already diagnosed with a condition either in the absence of treatment or in the setting of nontargeted standard treatment; as "predictive markers," which are predictors of drug response to mechanism-based targeted therapies (Pepe et al. 2008; Mandrekar and Sargent 2009); and as modulatable surrogate endpoints for key clinical outcomes (Fleming 2005) (Fig. 3.1). This paper will focus primarily on biomarkers in their application to screening and as surrogate endpoints in clinical prevention trials. Screening markers detect cancer prior to clinical presentation, leading to early detection that presumably results in improved outcomes. Surrogate endpoint biomarkers substitute for clinical endpoints, which assess a meaningful quality of patient health. An important caveat to this categorization of biomarkers is that in actual clinical applications a given biomarker may serve multiple purposes, as for example a biomarker that not only establishes increased risk of disease but is also modulatable and can therefore be used as a surrogate of clinical outcome.

In cancer the entities that often serve as biomarkers consist of physical material derived from biologic specimens from a variety of sources: tumor tissue itself; normal tissue associated with the tissue type of the tumor; or accessible nontumor tissue or secretions. The choice of specimen type depends on the planned biomarker application. The biomarker embodies a trait or a signature of traits that is associated with the cancer-related outcome of interest, whether cancer occurrence, prognosis, or response to therapy (Mandrekar and Sargent 2009). The actual physical material in which the trait(s) is measured ranges from DNA (for genotype) to messenger RNA or protein (for gene expression) to tissue specimens (for histopathology), depending on the purpose for which the biomarker will be used. In addition, images of the original tissue of interest, such as mammograms, frequently serve as biomarkers, particularly for purposes of risk assessment, screening, and diagnosis (Fabian and Kimler 2007).

3.1.1 Screening Biomarkers for Early Detection

Development of biomarkers for early detection of cancer is premised on the notion that preclinical cancer, evident only following active screening, is expected to have a greater chance of being curable than the larger, symptomatic tumors that present without screening. This position has generated an enthusiasm for screening that is evident in a variety of cancer types. Markers like CEA (carcinoembryonic antigen) in colorectal cancer and PSA in prostate cancer correlate with disease but are not in the disease-generation pathways (Fleming

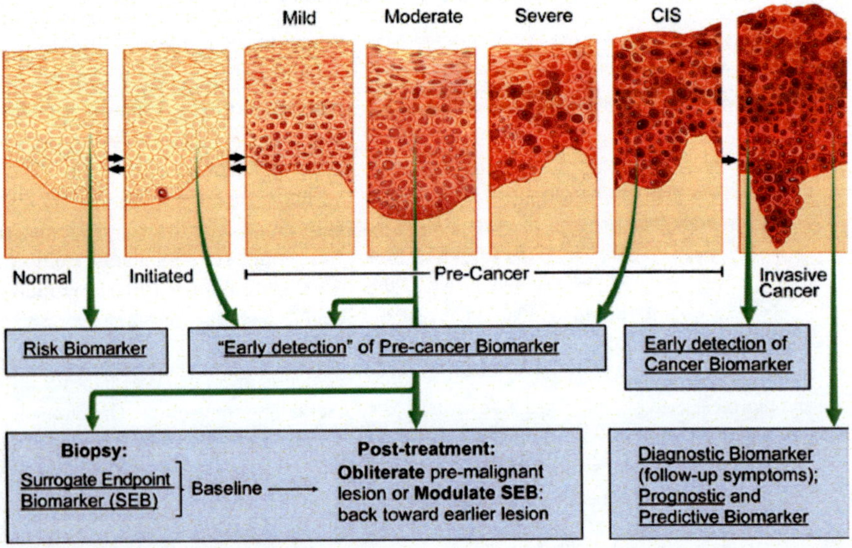

Fig. 3.1 Multiple purposes for which biomarkers are used. In cancer medicine biomarkers have been used for several purposes. Risk biomarkers reflect increased risk of a cancer type or subtype. "Early detection biomarkers" are used in screening of healthy but often increased-risk individuals for early stage cancers or for premalignant lesions. "Diagnostic biomarkers" are used to evaluate individuals with signs or symptoms for evidence of cancer. "Prognostic biomarkers" predict subsequent outcomes in patients already diagnosed with a condition either in the absence of treatment or in the setting of nontargeted standard treatment. "Predictive biomarkers" predict the likelihood of drug response, specifically the likelihood that a tumor will respond to a mechanism-based therapy targeted to that tumor. "Surrogate endpoint biomarkers (SEBs)" are used as substitutes for key clinical outcomes; modulation of SEBs in response to drug or other interventions should be in a direction that parallels the desired response of the clinical endpoint

2005). Research on CEA from the late 1960s to the early 1970s reported high sensitivity for CEA as a marker of colon cancer, but later analysis argued that an inadequate spectrum of patients was chosen to represent and compare diseased and nondiseased cases (Ransohoff and Feinstein 1978). Another highly controversial example is PSA which is widely used as a method for early detection of prostate cancer, even though it has never been validated as an effective screen in terms of decreased death due to this cancer. In contrast, an example of a good cancer biomarker of the development of cervical cancer is human papillomavirus (HPV). In-depth clinical insights tie the biomarker to the disease progression pathway, and empirical evidence shows that a high proportion of cervical cancers are linked to HPV infection (Schatzkin et al. 1990; zur Hausen 2000). High-throughput methods, including genomic and proteomic profiling, are expected to reveal many more potential markers in the coming years. In practical terms, the use of biomarkers in cancer prevention trials is most likely to be successful for cancer sites that are more accessible, such as the colon. Tissue, cells, and molecules are more readily obtained from tissues accessible through open tubes, and from organs that naturally generate secretions and excretions.

Early Detection Research Network (EDRN). In 2000, the National Cancer Institute (NCI)'s Division of Cancer Prevention established the EDRN to take a systematic approach to the development of cancer-screening biomarkers. The need for a systematic approach was considered especially pressing given the surge of data available with the growing use of gene-expression microarrays, proteomics, and other large-scale molecular techniques. The EDRN focuses on the discovery and validation of biomarkers for the early detection of cancer via noninvasive approaches. The research network includes laboratories developing biomarkers, laboratories validating biomarkers, clinical repositories, and population-screening programs. Such collaboration is intended to promote efficiency and rigor in research. By analogy to the clinical phases of testing a new drug, a five-phased approach to developing biomarkers for early detection of cancer has been proposed (Pepe et al. 2001). The first step includes discovery and exploratory studies; the second is validation to demonstrate the sensitivity and specificity of a biomarker in distinguishing people with cancer; the third is to test whether a biomarker can detect patients who will develop a disease before it is clinically evident by testing against longitudinally collected tissue specimens; the fourth step is prospective screening; and the fifth step involves large population studies to determine the impact of screening on health outcomes (see Table 3.1) (Cancer Biomarkers Research Group 2008). Designs of clinical trials for evaluation of biomarkers at critical steps in this phased progression have been proposed (Pepe et al. 2008; Mandrekar and Sargent 2009).

Table 3.1 Biomarker development as a phased process (Pepe et al. 2001)

Phase	Focus	Description
Phase 1	Preclinical (in vitro, in vivo) Exploratory Studies	Discovery; this phase involves exploratory studies to identify potentially useful biomarkers.
Phase 2	Clinical Assay Development for Clinical Disease; Clinical Validation	Validation at a clinical level involves studying biomarkers to determine their ability to distinguish between people with cancer and those without.
Phase 3	Retrospective Longitudinal and Repository Studies	Determines the capacity of a biomarker to detect disease before it presents clinically (preclinical disease) by testing the marker against tissues collected longitudinally from research cohorts. A "screen positive" rule is defined.
Phase 4	Prospective Screening Studies	Prospective screening studies determine the operating characteristics/performance of the biomarker screening test in large populations. These studies are used to determine the detection rate and the false referral rate.
Phase 5	Cancer Control Studies	Suggests the penultimate period in which large-scale population studies evaluate both the role of a biomarker for cancer detection and its overall screening impact, i.e. whether screening reduces the burden of cancer on the population.

EDRN researchers are attempting to circumvent a common pitfall of biomarker discovery – finding markers that reflect not the disease state but rather the differences in the way specimens were collected, as for example because of differences in study populations, methods of collection, or storage conditions across sets of biospecimens (Ransohoff and Gourlay 2010). To expedite biomarker development, the EDRN is developing standard specimen reference sets. The EDRN defines biomarkers as substances found in the blood, body fluids, or tissue that show the risk or presence of disease before cancer has progressed in the body. This definition excludes some promising candidate biomarkers, notably attributes that can be assessed through imaging, such as mammographic breast density, which is a promising marker for breast cancer (Fabian and Kimler 2006). The EDRN criteria for valid biomarkers are that they are reliable and repeatable in testing, sensitive and specific, quantitative, readily obtained by noninvasive methods, part of the causal pathway for disease, capable of being modulated by chemopreventive agents, and have high predictive value for clinical disease.

3.1.2 Biomarkers as Surrogate Endpoints in Cancer Prevention Trials

"A surrogate endpoint, or "marker", is a laboratory measurement or physical sign that is used in therapeutic trials as a substitute for a clinically meaningful endpoint that is a direct measure of how a patient feels, functions or survives, and is expected to predict the effect of the therapy." (Federal Register referenced in: [Schatzkin and Gail 2002]). In other words, biological markers that correlate with clinical efficacy endpoints can potentially be used as alternatives, i.e., surrogates, for the clinical endpoints of interest (Fleming 2005). Such surrogate endpoint biomarkers (SEBs) are potentially valuable in several ways. The most direct motivation for using them is their offer of greater efficiency in clinical studies. Compared to clinical endpoints, biomarkers may be more readily quantifiable, more easily assessed, and respond more quickly to medical interventions, allowing for the generation of useful results from studies that last a shorter time. Studies employing SEBs may require smaller numbers of study participants. As a result, SEBs can potentially reduce the duration, size and cost of clinical studies (Schatzkin and Gail 2002).

In this manner, the use of biomarkers is particularly promising in attempting to translate knowledge from basic research into clinical use. Assessing the response of biomarkers should allow for relatively rapid feedback as to whether an intervention is worth testing more definitively in a larger trial with clinical endpoints. Thus, using biomarkers in phase 2 trials can inform the prioritization of phase 3 trials (Fleming and DeMets 1996). Ultimately, the hope is that biomarkers that qualify as SEBs will aid in regulatory agencies' review and approval of new therapeutics. Smaller trials and faster decisions promise greater progress in achieving more individualized medical care. The use of SEBs can also lead to faster dose selection of new therapeutics. During this process, a negative predictive value is just as important as positive results; if an agent will fail, it is best for it to fail early, in an SEB-based trial, to expedite potentially more promising research. A hierarchy of outcome measures for SEB development has been proposed to ensure that progression of a candidate SEB to the level of an accepted substitute for the clinical outcome of interest is closely monitored (Fleming 2005).

Surrogate endpoint biomarkers in cancer prevention. SEBs offer particular promise for conducting trials involving the testing of potential chemopreventive agents where the clinical outcomes of interest, cancer incidence, and especially cancer-associated mortality, are rare events. The long latency of many forms of cancer can be a practical obstacle to showing that a chemopreventive strategy is indeed effective. Yet, the same protracted premalignant phase also provides an opportunity to intervene in order to avert progression to invasive cancer. SEBs in this prevention context should accurately reflect an agent's cancer-reducing effect by being modulated in a direction consistent with a reduction in carcinogenic activity (Fig. 3.1). Ideal surrogate endpoints should reliably predict clinical benefits, be easily and reliably quantified, and their modulation should not have toxic effects. The view of cancer as a disease of genetic progression supports the idea that molecular biomarkers should succeed as surrogate endpoints (Kelloff et al. 2006). Reducing progression of early premalignant lesions could benefit patients not only by reducing their risk of cancer and of death from cancer but also by reducing their need for invasive diagnostic procedures. Beyond their role as surrogates for true clinical endpoints, biomarkers can serve additional functions in prevention trials. Biomarkers can be used to help stratify individuals according to their risk of cancer and facilitate the selection of at-risk individuals for chemoprevention studies and ultimately for chemopreventive agent use.

To be useful as surrogate endpoints in cancer prevention trials, biomarkers should have a few key features. They must be subject to modulation. They should be reproducibly measured using minimally invasive techniques (Fabian et al. 2005). They should not vary greatly within individuals over the course of normal physiologic processes. A biomarker should have a high positive predictive value, so that a positive result with a biomarker assay reflects a high probability of a biological condition (Schatzkin et al. 1990). Biomarkers should reflect knowledge of underlying biological processes, validated by empirical evidence (Fleming 2005).

Reasons for Caution in the Use of Biomarkers as Surrogate Endpoints. To be used as reliable surrogate endpoints, biomarkers need to be validated. The biomarker development pipeline begins with identification, followed by initial evaluation as a reproducible laboratory test, and continues through to definitive clinical validation (Baker 2009). Initially, a biomarker should be chosen for clinically and biologically logical reasons. It is then tested at the laboratory level to show that it can be reliably isolated and measured. To be validated as a surrogate marker, biomarkers should be tested in large-scale, prospective clinical trials, with randomized subjects to avoid bias. The biomarker should be shown to be modulated in parallel to the modulation of a conventional clinical endpoint. This phase of SEB development, in which validation of the biomarker takes place within the context of clinical trials that contain conventional clinical endpoints against which the biomarker can be adjudicated, is critical. This would show the Food and Drug Administration Food and Drug Administration (FDA) that a biomarker is truly robust and useful. Through the process of validation, the sensitivity, specificity, and reproducibility of a biomarker's relationship with health outcomes should be measured (Wagner 2002). This is a high bar to cross, and has yet to be achieved in the context of cancer research.

A systematic approach to biomarker discovery and validation should help avoid many of the potential pitfalls of biomarker use. Biomarkers can have a complicated relationship with a disease (Fleming and DeMets 1996). A disease process can affect clinical outcomes through pathways that do not involve a proposed marker, and a treatment intervention may affect a marker through pathways that are independent of the disease process, in ways that are unintended and unrecognized (Fleming 2005; Schatzkin and Gail 2002; Fleming and DeMets 1996). Because of these complex interrelationships, such as the presence of a potential surrogate biomarker in a pathway separate from the one leading to the clinical outcome of interest, SEB modulation can occur in ways that show associations with the clinical endpoint but do not reflect true clinical benefits. In the absence of definitive validation of biomarkers in large-scale, prospective clinical trials, biomarkers should not be used as surrogate endpoints in phase 3 clinical trials. They can, however, be useful in phase 2 trials to suggest whether an intervention is promising and deserves further study.

Biomarkers in chemoprevention agent development. The complexity of the molecular origins of cancer presents a hurdle to the development of biomarkers for chemoprevention, both for purposes of surrogate endpoints and as targets of pharmaceutical interventions. Research on chemoprevention as well as cancer treatment has focused on targets in signal transduction pathways, especially growth factors and their receptors. Regulation of these pathways is complex, and inhibiting one target in a pathway may be ineffective or lead to unexpected side effects. These shortcomings may be mitigated by genomic and proteomic studies that take a comprehensive view of the effects of inhibiting a target. Not only are genomic and proteomic profiling methods expected to reveal many more potential markers for screening, but biomarkers emerging from these high throughput technologies, when linked to the pathophysiology of a disease, should provide a rational basis for choosing compounds for therapeutic testing. Using biomarkers grounded in an understanding of underlying biological mechanisms can clarify how interventions affect these mechanisms. Furthermore, systems approaches, including pathway analysis, which treat entire systems as biomarkers should also help in the design of chemopreventive strategies directed at multiple targets and pathways, and thereby more rationally affect molecular networks (Kelloff et al. 2006).

Because the intended population for a chemopreventive agent is essentially healthy, although at increased cancer risk, and may be exposed to the preventive intervention for many years, it is extremely important to determine the long-term risks and benefits of an intervention intended to prevent cancer.

Since 1992, the FDA has allowed the accelerated approval of drugs in studies that use biomarkers as surrogate endpoints, when the biomarkers are reasonably likely to predict clinical benefit based on an aggregation of statistical reasoning and clinical insight (Fleming 2005). After accelerated approval, drug manufacturers are expected to complete trials showing tangible clinical benefit. However, the FDA-mandated follow-up trials have been slow to occur and suffer from lack of participation in part because of availability of agents outside the setting of clinical trials. Thus, drugs have stayed on the market even if on further testing they failed to demonstrate substantial benefit (Fleming 2005).

3.2 Breast Precancer and Cancer Prevention

Epidemiologic data have historically offered a source of ideas for generating hypotheses regarding biomarkers as well as possible chemopreventive therapies (Schatzkin et al. 1990). For example, multiple epidemiological studies revealed an association of estrogen with breast cancer incidence. Models, like the Gail model, that are based on data from observational studies, in this case the case–control data from the Breast Cancer Detection Demonstration Project (Gail et al. 1989), predict breast cancer risk in populations that undergo regular screening. Yet, these models don't accurately predict individual risk (Fabian and Kimler 2007). Selective biomarkers may improve upon the ability of risk models to predict breast cancer risk in individuals. Biomarkers of this nature include genetic mutations such as those in the *BRCA1* and *BRCA2* genes. Mammographic density is also being explored as a potential marker of individual cancer risk (Tice et al.

2008). However, beyond risk, a need exists for biomarkers that are modulated in response to potential preventive interventions and can serve as surrogates for clinical endpoints in breast cancer chemoprevention trials. Biomarkers that are associated not only with increased risk but have also been used as surrogate response endpoints for breast cancer prevention studies include mammographic breast density, intraepithelial neoplasia (IEN) or cell proliferation, and molecular markers such as Ki-67, a marker of proliferation, serum IGF (insulin-like growth factor)-1 and the ratio of IGF-1 to the IGF binding protein (IGFBP)-3, and the estrogen receptor (ER) (Fabian and Kimler 2007; Kelloff et al. 2006).

IEN refers to lesions showing morphologic changes ranging from simple hyperplasia in the setting of an unfolded lobule through progressively abnormal looking cellular architecture to the malignant-appearing cells of the immediately preinvasive ductal carcinoma in situ (DCIS). The common feature in all IEN lesions is confinement of the abnormal tissue within boundaries of the basement membrane, in the case of breast tissue within the ducts or lobules; these are noninvasive lesions. Considerable attention has been given to the potential of IEN as a biomarker of risk and as a target of preventive intervention, but this type of preinvasive lesion might also serve as an SEB-based biomarker (Fabian and Kimler 2007; Kelloff et al. 2006). In one example, the risk of benign breast disease of various types, including IEN, was reduced with tamoxifen compared to placebo in the Breast Cancer Prevention Trial (BCPT) conducted by the National Cancer Institute (NCI) and the National Surgical Adjuvant Breast and Bowel Project (NSABP) (Fisher et al. 1998; Tan-Chiu et al. 2003). An important point to remember, however, is that although specific subtypes of IEN do correlate with increased risk and IEN in general has potential for use as a biomarker in chemoprevention trials (see below), IEN has not yet been validated as a biomarker for most of its proposed applications.

In another example of potentially useful SEBs, the recent surge in our understanding of epigenetic changes that are associated with cancer has offered a resource for molecular modifications that can be utilized as biomarkers. Certain modifications, such as methylated tumor suppressor genes individually or in designated panels, have been investigated as biomarkers for early detection and response (Fabian and Kimler 2007; Fackler et al. 2004; Lewis et al. 2005). As an example, hypermethylation of the genes *RASSF1a*, *HIN1*, and *Cyclin D2* are consistently associated with breast cancer, with high specificity but low sensitivity (Wang and Srivastava 2010). A reasonable approach to using these markers would be to pair a panel of methylated genes (high specificity/low sensitivity) with cytology (low specificity/high sensitivity) to produce a potential early detection strategy for asymptomatic women (Cancer Biomarkers Research Group 2008).

Finally, mention should be made of ongoing investigations that are utilizing biomarkers based on high-throughput technologies such as expression arrays (Fabian and Kimler 2007). In addition to revealing previously undetected individual molecular changes with potential to serve as biomarkers, such systems-level approaches give insight into the actual molecular pathways that are involved in carcinogenesis.

Phase 2 trials, which are often randomized, double-blind, placebo-controlled and typically enroll high-risk patients for 6–12 months, utilize biomarker endpoints. In addition, phase 1A trials may measure the effects of different doses of a drug on modulatable biomarkers in small sets of women. In breast cancer treatment research, a common phase 1A trial model is the presurgical design in which patients with DCIS or a small invasive cancer are given one of several doses of a drug or a placebo over the course of the few weeks between a biopsy that confirms the presence of disease and follow-up definitive surgery. A proliferation marker, typically Ki-67, is most often used as a surrogate endpoint for treatment efficacy. This method suffers from several difficulties. For example, Ki-67 levels vary in different parts of a tumor; in premenopausal women, there may be confounding effects in different phases of the menstrual cycle; or confounding effects may arise from tissue reaction to injury (Fabian et al. 2005).

3.2.1 Ductal Carcinoma In situ

Clarification of the prognosis of DCIS poses a major challenge to ongoing research efforts. The natural history of DCIS is not well understood because the lesion is usually excised surgically once discovered. Furthermore, the definition and classification of DCIS have become broader over time as widespread use of imaging modalities, such as mammography, has enabled the detection of ever-smaller forms of disease. DCIS incidence in the United States increased more than sevenfold from 1973 into the late 1990s, tracking with the increase in rates of mammographic screening (Allred et al. 2009). The most aggressive form of DCIS has central necrosis and microcalcifications. The average tumor size is slightly more than 1 cm. The invasive potential of DCIS varies among patients, as do its recurrence potential and response to treatment. The progression of benign cell proliferation into invasive disease can be rapid or occur very slowly. A better understanding of these differences in DCIS is necessary in order to determine which lesions require aggressive treatment and which can be adequately treated by simple surgical removal.

Thus, improvement is needed in the diagnostic accuracy and reproducibility of DCIS classifications and grading schemes. Arguments in favor of treating DCIS as an inevitable precursor to invasive cancer include the fact that DCIS cells are highly similar at the cellular and molecular levels to those of invasive breast cancer (IBC) and that nearly all IBC is found intermingled with DCIS. Yet, it is not yet known what proportion of DCIS actually would progress to IBC. Thus, although generally regarded as a target of treatment, DCIS itself can be thought of as a biomarker of breast cancer risk; DCIS shares risk factors with invasive breast cancer and is a strong predictor of future IBC, especially if it is not completely excised.

A great benefit could derive from the identification of prognostic biomarkers that occur in association with cases of DCIS that pose the highest risk of progression. To this end, a deeper understanding of the molecular mechanisms of invasion should not only provide a source of potential biomarkers but should also allow better prognostic insight and lead to new therapeutic strategies (Allred et al. 2009). Numerous studies have attempted to identify molecular factors in DCIS that predict the risk of invasive progression. Candidate markers include COX2 (cyclooxygenase 2), S100A7 and CD10, but no markers have been consistently able to predict the risk of invasive progression. No molecular markers other than hormone receptors and HER2 (human epidermal growth factor receptor 2) have proven to be better than the existing morphological grading and classification systems (Polyak 2009). Comprehensive studies of the genome, proteome, and epigenome in both the tumor epithelium and stromal environment may identify key events in tumor progression. DCIS subtypes appear to be genetically distinct: similar within the same woman and differing across women. In the future, gene expression profiling could help distinguish latent from potentially invasive forms of the condition (Fabian et al. 2005).

3.2.2 Tissue Stroma and Mammographic Density

Medical researchers are becoming increasingly aware of the importance of stromal biology in the development of breast cancer. The stroma is the supporting network of connective tissue in the breast. Recent research has shown that stromal cells cooperate with tumor cells to allow invasion (Ronnov-Jessen and Bissell 2009). The mechanisms of these epithelial–stromal interactions are the focus of ongoing investigations. A deeper understanding of the cellular and molecular mechanisms that undergird the interaction will hopefully suggest possible biomarkers. Research should clarify how characteristics of the stroma – as well as characteristics of tumor cells – should guide treatment choices. In essence, stromal attributes might well serve as risk and surrogate endpoint biomarkers.

Mammographic breast density is a well-established risk factor for breast cancer (Tice et al. 2008; Chen et al. 2006) and a modulatable biomarker. It reflects the relative amounts of stroma, fluid, and epithelium compared to fat in a breast (Fabian and Kimler 2007). But not all breast density is equivalent. Signaling from adjacent cells appears to be important in the development of invasive breast cancer, but as yet no methods exist to distinguish stromal cells that drive invasiveness from those that don't. More precise ways to interpret breast density, such as smaller-scale or even molecular-scale imaging, could clarify when breast density poses a risk. The usefulness of breast density as a surrogate endpoint marker is seen in its response to tamoxifen and other drugs that reduce the risk of estrogen-responsive breast cancer (Chow et al. 2000; Freedman et al. 2001; Cuzick et al. 2004; Eng-Wong et al. 2008); these drugs have been shown to reduce mammographic breast density. Conversely, mammographic breast density tends to increase upon estrogen exposure, for example, through hormone replacement therapy (Chlebowski and McTiernan 2003).

Blood levels of IGF-1 and its ratio to IGFBP-3 are molecular markers that correlate with breast density and estrogen exposure. Serum IGF-1 and the ratio of IGF-1 to IGFBP-3, which have been studied for use as SEBs for response to preventive interventions, are now undergoing assessment for early detection (Cancer Biomarkers Research Group 2008).

3.2.3 Biomarkers, ER-Positive Breast Cancer, and Breast Cancer Prevention Trials

Currently, the only FDA-approved drugs for preventing breast cancer target cancers that respond to estrogen (ER-positive, ER+breast cancers). No strategies have yet been validated for tumors that don't respond to estrogen (ER-negative, ER- breast cancers). Selective estrogen receptor modulators (SERMs) have the longest pedigree as a pharmaceutical approach for preventing ER+breast cancer. The SERM tamoxifen is FDA-approved to reduce the risk of ER+breast cancer and DCIS in women at increased risk of breast cancer. Another SERM, raloxifene (Eng-Wong 2004), has also been FDA-approved for decreasing the risk of first primary breast cancers in high-risk women, although only in postmenopausal women. In the NCI/NSABP's Breast Cancer Prevention Trial (BCPT), tamoxifen reduced the risks of ER+tumors and fractures resulting from osteoporosis, cutting the relative risk from breast cancer by nearly 50% (Fisher et al. 1998, 2005). In the follow-up Study of Tamoxifen and Raloxifene (STAR), another large phase 3 NCI-sponsored/NSABP-run trial comparing the relative effectiveness and safety of these two SERMs, the osteoporosis drug raloxifene proved to be as effective as tamoxifen in reducing the risk of invasive breast cancer in postmenopausal women and resulted in fewer side effects (Vogel et al. 2010). Interestingly, even those who do not show favorable biomarker modulation in response to tamoxifen can still benefit from the treatment; the observed benefit is greater than would be expected from the modulation of biomarkers including mammographic density (Fabian et al. 2005).

Arzoxifene is another SERM. In a phase 1 evaluation, arzoxifene was given to women between biopsy and re-excision. In addition to analyzing tumor tissue for modulation of biomarkers, specifically the proliferation marker Ki-67, serum collected before and after the arzoxifene intervention was tested for the levels of various hormones and growth factors. These hormones and growth factors, including sex hormones, IGF-1 and IGF-1:IGFBP-3 ratio, also served as surrogate endpoint biomarkers (Fabian et al. 2004). Reduction in the proportion of tumor cells expressing Ki-67 after short-term tamoxifen treatment has been shown to correlate with longer-term clinical response in women with breast cancer.

The toxicity of SERMs, particularly the increased risk of endometrial cancer with tamoxifen and the increase in thromboembolic disease with tamoxifen and raloxifene, have instigated a search for antiestrogens that are equally effective and lack these unacceptable side effects. As an alternative to the use of SERMs, aromatase inhibitors aromatase inhibitor (AIs), which almost completely inhibit estrogen production, are being evaluated as chemopreventive agents in postmenopausal women at high risk of breast cancer. Two large phase 3 breast cancer prevention trials evaluating the AIs anastrozole and exemestane are ongoing (Cuzick 2005; Goss et al. 2007). In addition, a phase 2 study of postmenopausal women at high risk of breast cancer who were taking hormone replacement therapy (HRT) assessed the effect of the AI letrozole on the biomarker Ki-67 in breast tissue obtained by random periareolar fine needle aspiration (RPFNA, see below). Letrozole treatment reduced this proliferation marker by 66%. This change was associated with reduced cellular abnormalities as assessed by karyometry but was not associated with any improvement in cytomorphology (Frank et al. 2009). Previous research has linked Ki-67 expression to a higher risk of breast cancer and lower chance of survival (de Azambuja et al. 2007). Clearly, more studies are needed to validate potentially meaningful combinations of informative markers. Karyometry could serve as a marker that integrates information about genetic abnormalities into a useful global biomarker in cancer cells.

The validation of any biomarker or combination of biomarkers as measures of the efficacy of chemopreventive strategies in breast cancer will require that they be correlated with long-term clinical outcomes. The reduction in risk of benign breast disease, including IEN, with tamoxifen in the BCPT (see above) offers an example of this approach. Similarly, the International Breast Intervention Study (IBIS)-1 trial, another of the four major studies comparing tamoxifen to placebo for prevention of breast cancer (Cuzick et al. 2003), also documented a reduction in mammographic density in women who took tamoxifen (Cuzick et al. 2004). In an ongoing phase 3 trial by the same group, the International Breast Intervention Study IBIS-II trial, biomarkers have been incorporated prospectively into the study design. International Breast Intervention Study IBIS-II, which is comparing the AI, anastrozole, to placebo for preventive efficacy, includes increased mammographic density as an eligibility criterion of high risk for entry onto the trial and a supplementary study of hormone levels in serum (Cuzick 2005, 2008).

3.2.4 Biomarkers and Estrogen Receptor-Negative Breast Cancers

Targeted interventions do not exist for estrogen receptor-negative (ER-) tumors, and there is a need for phase 2 trials of preventive drugs or food compounds addressing prevention of these cancers. Biomarker discovery may help in the development of agents for preventing ER- breast cancers. Potential biomarkers for use in trials evaluating these agents include markers of proliferation such as MiB2, markers of apoptosis and angiogenesis, and TGFβ type II receptor. Promising agents include tyrosine kinase inhibitors, retinoid-like compounds, statins, COX2 inhibitors, and farnesyl transferase inhibitors (Li and Brown 2009). ER- breast cancer was found to be less prevalent among statin users, with a retrospective cohort analysis showing that breast cancer patients who had taken statins had proportionately fewer hormone receptor-negative tumors (Kumar et al. 2008). This suggested a comprehensive strategy for preventing breast cancer by combining statins with agents that prevent ER+cancer – SERMs or aromatase inhibitors.

An important subset of ER- tumors are the triple negative breast cancers, which lack estrogen receptor, progesterone receptor, and HER2. Given their triple negativity, these tumors do not respond to available targeted therapies, whether herceptin or hormone antagonists. The majority of *BRCA1*-associated breast cancers are triple negative (Atchley et al. 2008; Anders and Carey 2008). A study in a mouse model with a *BRCA1*-mutation showed that tamoxifen did not protect against mammary cancer and in fact increased its incidence (Jones et al. 2005). However, drugs that hold promise for this subgroup of cancers are the poly(ADP-ribose) polymerase (PARP) inhibitors. PARP is an enzyme involved in the repair of DNA single-strand breaks. Inhibition of PARP leads to failure to repair single-strand breaks, which can now progress to double-strand breaks. *BRCA1* and *BRCA2* are important for the repair of DNA double-strand breaks (Boulton 2006). In cells that have BRCA1 or BRCA2 dysfunction, such double-strand breaks cannot be repaired. Hence, these cells are profoundly sensitive to the inhibition of PARP enzyme activity, resulting in cell cycle arrest and apoptosis (Farmer et al. 2005). Olaparib, an orally active PARP inhibitor, was shown to reduce the presence of tumors, as evaluated by serum tumor markers or radiology, in patients with *BRCA1* or *BRCA2* mutations who had breast, ovarian, or prostate cancer, with few adverse effects (Fong et al. 2009). A theoretical rationale suggests that PARP inhibitors would work more broadly in ER- breast cancer (Natrajan et al. 2010). PARP inhibitors are therefore also being investigated as preventive agents for ER- breast cancer in women other than *BRCA1/2*-mutation carriers.

3.2.5 Access to Breast Tissue for Biomarker Evaluation

In order to obtain breast epithelial cells to gauge morphology or the presence of certain biomarkers by the least invasive approaches possible, methods in use include obtaining nipple aspirate fluid, ductal lavage, RPFNA, and random and directed core needle biopsies (Fabian et al. 2005). RPFNA, because of its cost-effectiveness and efficiency in obtaining adequate amounts of sample, has proven to be the most practical option for tissue acquisition in breast cancer prevention trials (Arun et al. 2007). As a result, RPFNA is the most commonly used method of cell acquisition in phase 2 chemoprevention trials that assess modulation of breast cell proliferation in high-risk individuals. In such trials IEN may be used as a marker of risk. Atypical ductal hyperplasia, a subtype of IEN, often shares molecular and genetic changes with lesions along the IEN spectrum, including DCIS, as well as with invasive breast cancer (Fabian et al. 2005; Boecker et al. 2002). This commonality of abnormalities at the molecular level argues for the use of morphological abnormality, or IEN, as a biomarker for breast cancer risk. However, hyperplasia observed in cells obtained by RPFNA has shown low sensitivity for detecting known cases of breast cancer; in other words, many cases of breast cancer would be missed if one diagnosed cancer based solely on the morphology of cells obtained by RPFNA. On the plus side, RFPNA readily yields enough cells for quantitative PCR analysis of 6–12 biomarkers (Fabian et al. 2005). Like mammographic breast density, IEN is an attractive biomarker for breast cancer risk; both are subject to modulation and therefore useful as surrogate endpoint biomarkers in both pre and postmenopausal women. However, both molecular and other markers can vary greatly over the course of the menstrual cycle in premenopausal women. In the future, morphologic and molecular markers may be combined for more effective risk stratification.

3.2.6 Biomarkers in Phase 2 Chemoprevention Trials

In addition to helping assess whether a preventive measure seems promising, biomarkers associated with breast cancer risk can be used to assign individual risk for purposes of selecting high-risk cohorts for prevention intervention trials. In a phase 2 chemoprevention trial of α-difluoromethylornithine (DFMO), subjects were selected on the basis of hyperplasia in cells obtained by RPFNA. Measured SEBs included: improvement in cytomorphology; molecular markers, including the expression of proliferating cell nuclear antigen (PCNA), p53, EGF receptor, and IGF-1:IGFBP-3 ratio; and mammographic breast density. The study also tracked subsequent breast cancer development (Fabian et al. 2002). No improvement in these measures was observed among women treated with DFMO.

A 2005 study (Kong et al. 2005) evaluated the effect of a potent RXR-selective retinoid, LGD1069 (Bexarotene), on COX2 expression. COX is involved in inflammation, and inhibitors of COX, such as aspirin and nonsteroidal anti-inflammatory drugs (NSAIDs), have been shown to prevent cancer in animal models. Retinoids are derivatives of vitamin A that inhibit the growth of several human cancer cell lines and suppress tumor formation in animals, but the use of retinoids has been limited in humans because of their toxicity. LGD1069 seemed promising because it bound selectively compared to other retinoids and was still observed to suppress COX2 expression. This suggested the possibility that LGD1069 could serve as a chemopreventive intervention for ER- breast cancer. Retinoids could, in theory, be used in combination with chemopreventive agents such as antiestrogens or COX2 inhibitors for prevention of a broader spectrum of breast cancer subtypes. The hope is that the use of combination strategies will increase the efficacy of chemoprevention treatments while minimizing their toxicity.

A recent study (Yang et al. 2010) sought to discover molecular pathways associated with increased mammographic breast density, based on the hypothesis that identifying those pathways could lead to targets for chemoprevention. The study compared breast tissue characteristics in women with high and low breast density using large-scale gene expression arrays as well as immunohistochemistry to analyze levels of ER-, PR, Ki-67, and COX2 expression. The study found differential expression in more than 70 genes and decreased TGFβ signaling in denser breast tissue. COX2 expression in stroma was found to be increased in denser breast tissue. TGFβ ligands are the only growth factors known to prevent the proliferation of mammary epithelial cells, and COX2 has been reported to inhibit TGFβ signaling. This study reinforced the notion that COX2 inhibition could be an important targeted mechanism for breast cancer prevention. Although COX2 inhibitors were once widely touted as promising agents for chemoprevention, fears of cardiovascular side effects associated with these agents (Drazen 2005) have curtailed interest in COX2 inhibitor chemoprevention studies in breast and other cancers. Yet, lower doses and modified schedules of drug administration with COX2 inhibitors could minimize cardiovascular side effects and improve life expectancy in those at high risk of breast or other cancers.

Another example of biomarkers that can serve in a variety of roles in phase 2 trials are IGF and the associated IGF-1:IGFBP-3 ratio. Because IGF levels are increased in many cancers while the levels of IGFBP-3, which inhibits IGF signaling, are decreased, and because SERMs and retinoids, which lower cell proliferation, also lower the IGF-1:IGFBP-3 ratio, the pathways associated with IGF are attractive targets for chemoprevention (Kelloff et al. 2006). In the long term, studies of breast cancer risk should move from identifying cellular anomalies based on cell morphology to defining anomalies by molecular attributes, preferably at the pathway level.

3.3 Prostate Cancer Prevention

3.3.1 PSA Screening and Early Detection of Prostate Cancer

Even more than with breast cancer, a pressing need exists for tests that can predict the malignant potential of prostate cancer cells. The reason is that PSA testing as a prostate cancer screen is widely used and a large proportion of prostate cancers detected in this manner are indolent and would likely never lead to death due to this disease, reflecting "overdiagnosis." Until recently, the American Cancer Society (ACS) recommended offering annual PSA testing beginning at the age of 50 years to men with a normal age-related risk of prostate cancer and starting at an earlier age for men at high risk. Yet, studies have shown that the use of PSA as a biomarker for early detection of prostate cancer does not appear to result in reduced prostate cancer mortality (Kelloff et al. 2006). To assess more definitively whether a number of cancer screening tests, including PSA screening, reduce death rates from cancer, NCI's Division of Cancer Prevention sponsored and ran the Prostate, Lung, Colorectal and Ovarian Cancer Screening Trial (PLCO) (Gohagan et al. 2000). From 1993 through 2001, the PLCO trial followed nearly 77,000 men at ten study centers, of whom half were randomly assigned to a group that offered annual PSA testing and half for observation. The incidence of prostate cancer diagnosis was 22% higher in the screened group, but prostate cancer mortality was no lower; in fact, the death rate was slightly higher in the group offered annual PSA screening (Andriole et al. 2009).

Currently, NCI, the US Preventive Services Task Force, and the ACS do not support routine testing for prostate cancer. A more specific form of prostate cancer detection than PSA testing is required. Panels of markers may offer a better solution for disease detection, predicting disease severity, choosing treatments, and monitoring response to therapies (Sardana et al. 2008).

3.3.2 Phase 3 Prostate Cancer Prevention Trials

Strategies for preventing prostate cancer have been tested in large clinical trials that measure the incidence of cancer as an endpoint. The NCI-sponsored/Southwest Oncology Group (SWOG)-run Prostate Cancer Prevention Trial

(PCPT) was a 7-year phase 3 trial that tested finasteride for its chemopreventive efficacy. Finasteride inhibits 5-alpha-reductase, the enzyme that converts testosterone to dihydrotestosterone (DHT), the biologically active metabolite important to prostate growth. Finasteride was already approved by the FDA to shrink benign hypertrophy of the prostate and to treat male-pattern baldness. The PCPT study of more than 18,000 men showed a 25% reduction in prostate cancer incidence in those who took finasteride, but the same group had a higher proportion of aggressive forms of prostate cancer (Thompson et al. 2003). Finasteride appeared to be more effective in preventing low-grade than high-grade tumors and apparently improved the detection of remaining high-grade cancer cells by shrinking overall prostate size (Lucia et al. 2007). The trial was not large enough to show any differences in prostate cancer-specific mortality between the finasteride and placebo arms. Despite these limitations, the reduction in number of prevalent prostate cancers can be seen as a substantial benefit because reducing the morbidity associated with treating prostate cancer is a clinically beneficial endpoint in itself (Kramer et al. 2009). In addition to the primary chemopreventive endpoint of the PCPT, data from men not treated with finasteride (placebo arm) indicated that biopsy-detected prostate cancer, including high-grade cancer, is not uncommon in men with PSA levels $\leq$4.0 ng/ml, the usual threshold for the "normal" range (Thompson et al. 2004). These observations further weaken arguments favoring PSA level as a specific screen for prostate cancer.

The Selenium and Vitamin E Cancer Prevention Trial (SELECT) is another large-scale, long-term NCI/SWOG-sponsored study that evaluated these two nutrients by means of a partial factorial design. The SELECT study did not reveal a reduction in prostate cancer incidence from the use of selenium or vitamin E supplements alone or in combination (Lippman et al. 2009). A great deal of discussion has ensued addressing the reasons for the absence of observed benefit from these two promising nutritional agents (Dunn et al. 2010). Large phase 3 trials like PCPT and SELECT are necessarily expensive, both in infrastructure costs and in the use of human resources. Using validated biomarkers as surrogate endpoints for cancer incidence could potentially avoid the need for large trials that might ultimately show no benefit from an intervention. Small, short-term studies of biomarker modulation could offer a more efficient way of evaluating potential preventive approaches, conserving resources for fewer large-scale, long-term trials that measure cancer incidence and severity.

3.3.3 Discovery of New Biomarkers for Early Detection of Prostate Cancer

The EDRN is engaged in efforts to find biomarkers for prostate cancer, including biomarkers for diagnosis and prognosis. In a promising lead, EDRN researchers have discovered the presence of recurrent gene fusions in prostate cancers (Kumar-Sinha et al. 2008). These fusions include chromosomal rearrangements that juxtapose the *TMPRSS2* (transmembrane protease, serine 2) promoter and the first non-coding exon of genes in the *ETS* (E-twenty six) family of oncogenes (*ETV1, ETV4,* (ETS translocation variant) and *ERG (ETS related gene)*). The majority of prostate cancers have these rearrangements, but they are not present in normal prostate cells. Furthermore, they have been shown to be partly responsible for transformation of normal to cancerous cells (Tomlins et al. 2005). The gene fusions appear to define distinct classes of prostate cancer that bear on the prognosis and best treatment choices for particular patients (Tomlins et al. 2005). Among fusion-negative prostate cancers, a proportion exhibit over-expression of the biomarker SPINK1, which is a predictor of aggressive prostate cancer (Tomlins et al. 2008). The potential of both biomarkers for noninvasive early detection is evident in the fact that RNA transcripts reflecting the *TMPRSS2-ETS* gene fusion rearrangements and *SPINK1* overexpression have been detected in urine of men with the respective type of prostate cancer (Laxman et al. 2008). In another approach, metabolomic profiling also showed a possible role of sarcosine in prostate cancer progression (Sreekumar et al. 2009).

Other candidate biomarkers for prostate cancer early detection and prognosis include more nuanced ways of measuring PSA, such as PSA change over time ("PSA velocity"); levels of human kallikrein-related peptidase 2, a secreted protease from the same gene family as PSA; prostate-specific membrane antigen (PSMA); other kallikreins, several of which are produced at relatively high concentrations in the prostate; prostate cancer antigen 3 (PCA3), a noncoding RNA produced in the prostate and overproduced in prostate cancer; and other proteins that are expressed in the prostate and overexpressed in prostate cancer cells. Genomic expression and proteomic patterns could lead to the identification of multiple markers that could be used collectively to more fully characterize types of prostate cancers (Sardana et al. 2008).

Finding better biomarkers as surrogate endpoints for prostate cancer would enable short-term trials for measuring the effects of drugs or supplements on disease incidence. For example, during the few weeks that elapse between the taking of a prostate biopsy that detects cancer cells and the follow-up definitive surgery that removes the prostate, potential preventive agents can be administered and modulation of surrogate endpoint biomarkers can be monitored as responses to the interventions. In one such study that randomized 161 prostate cancer patients to a usual diet, a flaxseed-supplemented diet, a low-fat diet, or a flaxseed-supplemented, low-fat diet for an average of 30 days between biopsy and definitive prostate surgery, proliferation rates as measured by Ki-67 positivity were significantly lower ($P<0.002$) in the flaxseed arms (Demark-Wahnefried et al. 2008). Additional promising agents for prostate cancer prevention include antioxidants, SERMs, NSAIDs, soy isoflavones, and statins (Kelloff et al. 2006).

3.4 Colorectal Cancer Prevention

Colorectal cancer is a form of disease where screening and simultaneous removal of suspicious lesions, as done during colonoscopies, is a very effective way to prevent or treat early cancer. Adenomatous polyps can be considered surrogate endpoints for colorectal cancer. These polyps, which typically linger for a long time in the body before becoming cancerous, are removed during colonoscopies. In this manner, colonoscopies are estimated to be able to prevent 80% of colorectal cancers (Itzkowitz 2009). Similarly, removal of advanced adenomas containing noninvasive or early-stage malignant lesions can prevent advancement to later stages. But colonoscopies are invasive procedures, and despite their efficacy in preventing cancer, less than 40% of people over 50 undergo screening for colorectal cancer (Imperiale et al. 2004). Less invasive tests, such as analysis of stool DNA, are promising as alternative or supplementary approaches to early colorectal cancer detection. The molecular pathogenesis of colorectal cancer is relatively well defined, and DNA marker panels for purposes of early detection can be expanded or refined as knowledge about tumor biology evolves.

Aspirin and other nonsteroidal anti-inflammatory drugs have been associated with a reduced risk of colorectal cancer. In the Prevention of Colorectal Sporadic Adenomatous Polyps trial (Arber et al. 2006), participants who took the COX2 inhibitor celecoxib daily had a reduced risk of developing colorectal adenomas and especially advanced adenomas. However, NSAIDs and COX2 inhibitors have side effects and therefore haven't been recommended for long-term use to prevent cancer (Bertagnolli et al. 2006).

Combinations of drugs offer a promising strategy for prevention of cancer, potentially allowing the use of lower drug doses and more effectively preventing cancer. Meyskens et al. (2008) used two drugs in low doses – sulindac, an NSAID, and DFMO, which inhibits cells' synthesis of polyamines, molecules that have been associated with cell growth and cancer. Patients taking the two drugs, who had previously had adenomas removed, showed a 70% reduction in the recurrence of adenomas. The frequency of advanced adenomas was even more dramatically reduced. DFMO and sulindac affect separate pathways that drive cell proliferation. Before this trial, studies in rodents had suggested that a combination regimen of DFMO and an NSAID could have a beneficial effect (Meyskens and Gerner 1999).

Stool-based DNA testing offers a promising, noninvasive approach to early detection of precancerous lesions. Compared to fecal occult blood testing, stool-based DNA testing has several advantages: DNA testing does not require dietary or medication restrictions; appears to be more sensitive in detecting lesions; is better at detecting lesions located proximally in the colon; and offers the prospect of earlier diagnosis, detecting polyps before they have started to bleed (Schroy and Heeren 2005). DNA tests that target processes early in cancer development offer greater promise for preventing cancer. The first DNA markers used for colorectal cancer screening were chosen to detect existing cancers, whereas new panels of biomarkers are geared to detect earlier changes that occur in premalignant adenomas. These early detection biomarkers include aberrant methylation as well as sequence alterations in specific genes (Itzkowitz 2009). A diverse panel of markers can be used to accommodate the molecular heterogeneity of colorectal cancers (Ahlquist et al. 2008). Technical improvements, such as the use of stabilization buffers to better preserve DNA, better marker panels, and improved analysis methods promise to make stool-based DNA testing more sensitive and a good supplement to or substitute for colonoscopies (Ahlquist 2009).

Stool-based DNA testing even has the potential to detect gastrointestinal (GI) cancers much higher than the colon, such as cancers of the pancreas, stomach, and esophagus. Supracolonic GI cancers kill twice as many people in the United States as colorectal cancers, and most are diagnosed at a late stage with little chance for cure. Stool screening to detect a wide range of GI cancers could transform their treatment. Screening for cancer in multiple organs with a single, noninvasive test could also be very cost-effective and for the first time justify the screening of even uncommon cancers (Ahlquist 2009). For widespread clinical application, DNA marker panels need to be optimized and assays must be sensitive and specific. Algorithms should be developed to efficiently evaluate results so as to inform clinical decision making.

Among the current screening modalities is low dose computed tomography (CT)/CT colonography. While colonoscopy and flexible sigmoidoscopy are invasive, uncomfortable, and expensive, CT colonography, a new and less studied technology, is less invasive. Yet, colonography still requires a bowel preparation and follow-up colonoscopy with biopsy for suspicious lesions. The acceptability of the various colorectal cancer screening modalities among healthy people to whom they are directed was the subject of a recent NIH State-of-the-Science Conference (National Cancer Institute 2010).

3.5 Lung Cancer Prevention

Lung cancer is the leading cause of cancer death in the United States, accounting for more deaths than colon, breast, and prostate cancer combined.

Most cases of lung cancer are detected after the disease has spread, but when lung cancer is detected early, survival rates are much improved. Unfortunately, attempts to detect lung cancer early through chest X-rays and sputum cytology have historically been unsuccessful (Kelloff et al. 2006). Computerized tomography (CT) scans can detect nodules in the lung, but the high false positive rate and need for follow-up scans expose patients to unnecessary radiation, anxiety, and financial burdens. The NCI's Division of Cancer Prevention is currently conducting a prospective randomized trial, the National Lung Screening Trial (NLST), in 50,000 current and former smokers comparing spiral CT to standard chest X-rays to see if either test is superior at reducing deaths due to lung cancer (NLST 2010). A parallel effort has been implemented by the American College of Radiology Imaging Network.

3.5.1 Molecular Markers for Early Detection and Prognosis

The NCI-sponsored EDRN is attempting to identify biomarkers in blood or sputum for the early detection of lung cancer. One category of potential biomarker involves a particular type of epigenetic modification, the methylation status of the promoters of various genes, specifically tumor suppressor genes. Promoter methylation is associated with the silencing of gene expression, and aberrant gene expression and promoter methylation are commonly found during the development of lung cancer (Cancer Biomarkers Research Group 2008; Belinsky 2004; Belinsky et al. 2006). DNA methylation can be readily assessed by techniques based on the polymerase chain reaction (PCR). In one study, plasma and sputum from patients with abnormalities detected by means of CT scanning were examined for methylation of various genes. Four gene promoters (*CDH1, RASSF1A, p16,* and *MGMT*) exhibited methylation, and thus have potential as early detection markER-s (Cancer Biomarkers Research Group 2008). Only 4% of control patients in the study showed methylation in one gene, whereas methylation of at least one gene was seen in patients with nodules (30%), ground-glass opacities (GGOs; 32%), and cancerous tumors (48%). In sputum, methylation of at least one marker was found in only 6% of controls but was present in higher numbers in individuals with nodules (18%) and GGOs (41%). A follow-on study is using the same methods to investigate a panel of genes that includes *APC, Cyclin D2,* β-*Catenin, FHIT, Calcitonin-Related Peptide, DNA Methyltransferase,* and *Deleted in Colorectal Cancer (DCC).* Chromosomal instability is also associated with the development of lung cancer, and chromosomal abnormalities can be detected in smokers at high risk who do not yet have lung cancer (Cancer Biomarkers Research Group 2008; Jonsson et al. 2008). Chromosomal profiles and the methylation status of panels of relevant genes could serve as biomarkers for early forms of lung cancer.

Although a validated early detection molecular marker has yet to be identified, progress has been made with additional, ongoing investigations using not only sputum and serum, but also exhaled air. A promising marker panel, currently being validated in a large, cross-sectional study, includes the serum markers for annexin 1, PGP9.5, and 14-3-3 theta proteins (Qiu et al. 2008). Previous studies have shown that annexin 1, 14-3-3 theta, and the lung cancer antigen LAMR1 are present in serum before the symptoms or diagnosis of lung cancer. A number of individual molecular markers have been linked to either lung cancer risk or prognosis. Markers of prognosis include growth regulators, particularly mutations in *K-ras* and over-expression of the epidermal growth factor receptor (EGFR); over-expression of proteins expressed primarily during cell division, such as Ki-67, proliferating cell nuclear antigen (PCNA), and the minichromosome maintenance protein (MCM2); the loss of inhibitors of cell proliferation, such as p53; and reduced expression of Bcl-2, an inhibitor of programmed cell death (Vourlekis and Szabo 2004). Integrating information from multiple markers could help increase the value of molecular findings in clinical practice.

3.5.2 Treating Nicotine Addiction

With 87% of lung cancer cases thought to be the consequence of smoking, one effective form of chemoprevention is to help smokers quit smoking or to help prevent relapse in former smokers. Antinicotine vaccines have been tested in phase 2 trials by at least three companies – Nabi Pharmaceuticals based in the United States, the Swiss company Cytos, and the United Kingdom's Xenova Group. The vaccines lead to the formation of antibodies against nicotine; the antibodies bind to nicotine in the blood stream and prevent nicotine from crossing into the brain. The end points that the phase 2 studies have assessed are reduced smoking and fewer cravings. The trials have also used biochemical measures of smoke intake, including concentrations of urinary cotinine, a metabolite of nicotine, and of NNAL (4-(N-nitrosomethylamino)-1-(3-pyridyl)-1-butanol), a metabolite of tobacco processing-associated nitrosamines (Hatsukami et al. 2005). A drug called varenicline marketed by Pfizer takes a slightly different approach to alleviating nicotine cravings. The drug binds to the nicotine receptor, preventing nicotine from activating the receptor. In addition to helping prevent lung cancer, drugs that break nicotine addiction can also help prevent the 30% of all cancer deaths that result from smoking.

3.5.3 Fluorescence Bronchoscopy

Fluorescence bronchoscopy has emerged in recent years as a technique for detecting lesions in individuals at high risk for lung cancer. The method uses differences in autofluorescence between normal and dysplastic tissues to detect abnormalities in the large airways. Because the method only reveals abnormalities in a small portion of the lung, it is not used widely to screen patients, but it can be helpful in research studies (Vourlekis and Szabo 2004). For example, fluorescence bronchoscopy can be useful in chemoprevention trials. Bronchial fluorescence was used as a surrogate end point in a phase 1 trial that assessed the potential of *myo*-inositol in preventing lung cancer (Lam et al. 2006). *myo*-Inositol is an isomer of glucose linked to cell signaling and found in a wide variety of foods, such as whole grains, fruit, and seeds. It was found to be safe and effective in promoting the regression of bronchial dysplasia in smokers at high risk for lung cancer. The substance also appears to have other health benefits and has been investigated as a treatment for psychiatric disorders and diabetic neuropathy. Unexpectedly, *myo*-inositol was also found to reduce blood pressure (Lam et al. 2006).

3.6 Conclusions

Many biomarkers are being actively investigated for potential application to various clinical purposes (Fig. 3.1, Table 3.2). Ideal biomarkers both for early detection of cancer and precancer and for use as surrogate endpoints in cancer prevention trials should be both easy to measure using noninvasive methods and readily quantifiable. Surrogate endpoint biomarkers should also be subject to modulation but consistent within

Table 3.2 Examples of biomarkers for various cancer sites

Name of biomarker	Type of biomarker (role played by biomarker)	Cellular activity represented by biomarker	Example of clinical trial or study using this biomarker/cancer site	Reference [reference to a trial or a review describing the biomarker]
Ki-67	Surrogate endpoint; risk prediction; prognosis	Cell proliferation	Letrozole trial/Breast cancer	(Fabian and Kimler 2007; Frank et al. 2009; de Azambuja et al. 2007)
HPV	Early detection	Viral infection	/Liver cancer	(Schatzkin et al. 1990; zur Hausen 2000)
BRCA1, BRCA2	Risk prediction	DNA repair	/Breast cancer, Ovarian cancer	(Boulton 2006)
Ratio of IGF-1 to IGFBP	Surrogate endpoint	Growth factor signaling	/Breast cancer	(Fabian et al. 2004)
Estrogen Receptor	Classification of disease; drug response	Cell response to growth signals	Breast Cancer Prevention Trial (BCPT); Study of Tamoxifen and Raloxifene (STAR)/Breast cancer	(Fisher et al. 1998) (Vogel et al. 2006)
Aberrant gene methylation	Early detection; drug response	Expression of genes involved in cancer development	/Breast cancer, Colorectal cancer	(Fabian and Kimler 2007; Fackler et al. 2004; Lewis et al. 2005; Itzkowitz 2009)
Mammographic breast density	Risk prediction; Surrogate endpoint	Stromal environment	NCI Breast Cancer Surveillance Consortium; Breast Cancer Detection Demonstration Project; International Breast Intervention Study (IBIS)-II/Breast cancer	(Fisher et al. 1998; Tice et al. 2008; Chen et al. 2006; Cuzick 2008)
SPINK1	Early detection, Diagnosis, prognosis	Invasion, possibly	Prostate cancer	(Tomlins et al. 2008, 2005)
Bronchial autofluorescence	Surrogate endpoint	Tissue lesion	*myo*-Inositol trial/Lung cancer	(Vourlekis and Szabo 2004; Lam et al. 2006)

individuals over normal physiologic processes, and they should reflect biological understanding of carcinogenic pathways. To be truly reliable, biomarkers need to be validated in the laboratory as repeatable tests and in the clinic as early detection or surrogate endpoint biomarkers; the latter process can take a great deal of time. In fact, no biomarkers have been clinically validated as surrogate endpoints, although many markers show promise. In order to be validated clinically, surrogate endpoint biomarkers should be followed within large-scale, randomized clinical trials, to assess whether the markers track with clinical outcomes. Such studies require a great investment of resources. Yet, once validated in the context of such studies, biomarkers could be used to circumvent these long-term, large-scale trials that are designed, but sometimes fail, to demonstrate the benefits of a clinical intervention. In addition to economizing on the extensive resources required for phase 3 trials, preliminary testing with validated surrogate biomarkers should direct resources away from unpromising trials. In the future, researchers may necessarily devote more attention to phase 2 trials, assessing changes in biomarkers in relatively small numbers of people over shorter periods of time. Adaptive trial designs also hold promise for circumventing large-scale phase 3 trials (Mandrekar and Sargent 2009). This is a statistically-based, flexible approach to clinical studies in which results obtained during a trial are incorporated into adaptation of the design of a study midstream. In order that smaller, shorter-term trials that conserve resources yield reliable conclusions and directions for future research, there is an urgent need to validate biomarkers in the laboratory and, even more so, at the clinical level.

Acknowledgements The authors thank Darrell Anderson and Paul Wagner for sharing their insights on biomarkers during the writing of the manuscript. We also thank Lydia Kibiuk for providing graphics expertise in the design of Fig. 3.1.

References

Ahlquist DA (2009) Next-generation stool DNA testing: expanding the scope. Gastroenterology 136:2068–2073

Ahlquist DA, Sargent DJ, Loprinzi CL, Levin TR, Rex DK, Ahnen DJ, Knigge K, Lance MP, Burgart LJ, Hamilton SR, Allison JE, Lawson MJ, Devens ME, Harrington JJ, Hillman SL (2008) Stool DNA and occult blood testing for screen detection of colorectal neoplasia. Ann Intern Med 149(441–50):W81

Allred DC (2009) Terminology, natural history, and taxonomy of ductal carcinoma in situ. NIH State-of-the-Science Conference: Diagnosis and Management of Ductal Carcinoma In Situ (DCIS). September 22–24, Bethesda, MD. NIH State-of-the-Science Conference: Diagnosis and Management of Ductal Carcinoma In Situ (DCIS). September 22–24, Bethesda, MD. http://consensus.nih.gov/2009/dcisstatement.htm. Accessed February 26, 2010

Anders C, Carey LA (2008) Understanding and treating triple-negative breast cancer. Oncology (Williston Park) 22:1233–1239

Andriole GL, Crawford ED, Grubb RL III, Buys SS, Chia D, Church TR, Fouad MN, Gelmann EP, Kvale PA, Reding DJ, Weissfeld JL, Yokochi LA, O'Brien B, Clapp JD, Rathmell JM, Riley TL, Hayes RB, Kramer BS, Izmirlian G, Miller AB, Pinsky PF, Prorok PC, Gohagan JK, Berg CD (2009) Mortality results from a randomized prostate-cancer screening trial. N Engl J Med 360:1310–1319

Arber N, Eagle CJ, Spicak J, Racz I, Dite P, Hajer J, Zavoral M, Lechuga MJ, Gerletti P, Tang J, Rosenstein RB, Macdonald K, Bhadra P, Fowler R, Wittes J, Zauber AG, Solomon SD, Levin B (2006) Celecoxib for the prevention of colorectal adenomatous polyps. N Engl J Med 355:885–895

Arun B, Valero V, Logan C, Broglio K, Rivera E, Brewster A, Yin G, Green M, Kuerer H, Gong Y, Browne D, Hortobagyi GN, Sneige N (2007) Comparison of ductal lavage and random periareolar fine needle aspiration as tissue acquisition methods in early breast cancer prevention trials. Clin Cancer Res 13:4943–4948

Atchley DP, Albarracin CT, Lopez A, Valero V, Amos CI, Gonzalez-Angulo AM, Hortobagyi GN, Arun BK (2008) Clinical and pathologic characteristics

of patients with BRCA-positive and BRCA-negative breast cancer. J Clin Oncol 26: 4282–4288
Baker SG (2009) Improving the biomarker pipeline to develop and evaluate cancer screening tests. J Natl Cancer Inst 101:1116–1119
Belinsky SA (2004) Gene-promoter hypermethylation as a biomarker in lung cancer. Nat Rev Cancer 4:707–717
Belinsky SA, Liechty KC, Gentry FD, Wolf HJ, Rogers J, Vu K, Haney J, Kennedy TC, Hirsch FR, Miller Y, Franklin WA, Herman JG, Baylin SB, Bunn PA, Byers T (2006) Promoter hypermethylation of multiple genes in sputum precedes lung cancer incidence in a high-risk cohort. Cancer Res 66:3338–3344
Bertagnolli MM, Eagle CJ, Zauber AG, Redston M, Solomon SD, Kim K, Tang J, Rosenstein RB, Wittes J, Corle D, Hess TM, Woloj GM, Boisserie F, Anderson WF, Viner JL, Bagheri D, Burn J, Chung DC, Dewar T, Foley TR, Hoffman N, Macrae F, Pruitt RE, Saltzman JR, Salzberg B, Sylwestrowicz T, Gordon GB, Hawk ET (2006) Celecoxib for the prevention of sporadic colorectal adenomas. N Engl J Med 355:873–884
Boecker W, Moll R, Dervan P, Buerger H, Poremba C, Diallo RI, Herbst H, Schmidt A, Lerch MM, Buchwalow IB (2002) Usual ductal hyperplasia of the breast is a committed stem (progenitor) cell lesion distinct from atypical ductal hyperplasia and ductal carcinoma in situ. J Pathol 198:458–467
Boulton SJ (2006) Cellular functions of the BRCA tumour-suppressor proteins. Biochem Soc Trans 34:633–645
Cancer Biomarkers Research Group (2008) EDRN fourth report: investing in translational research on biomarkers of early cancer and cancer risk. NIH Publication No. 07-6135, 1-126. 2008, Bethesda, MD, National Institutes of Health, National Cancer Institute. http://edrn.nci.nih.gov/docs/progress-reports/edrn_4th-report_200801.pdf. Accessed February 26, 2010
Chen J, Pee D, Ayyagari R, Graubard B, Schairer C, Byrne C, Benichou J, Gail MH (2006) Projecting absolute invasive breast cancer risk in white women with a model that includes mammographic density. J Natl Cancer Inst 98:1215–1226
Chlebowski RT, McTiernan A (2003) Biological significance of interventions that change breast density. J Natl Cancer Inst 95:4–5
Chow CK, Venzon D, Jones EC, Premkumar A, O'Shaughnessy J, Zujewski J (2000) Effect of tamoxifen on mammographic density. Cancer Epidemiol Biomarkers Prev 9:917–921
Cuzick J (2005) Aromatase inhibitors for breast cancer prevention. J Clin Oncol 23:1636–1643
Cuzick J (2008) IBIS II: a breast cancer prevention trial in postmenopausal women using the aromatase inhibitor anastrozole. Expert Rev Anticancer Ther 8:1377–1385
Cuzick J, Powles T, Veronesi U, Forbes J, Edwards R, Ashley S, Boyle P (2003) Overview of the main outcomes in breast-cancer prevention trials. Lancet 361:296–300
Cuzick J, Warwick J, Pinney E, Warren RM, Duffy SW (2004) Tamoxifen and breast density in women at increased risk of breast cancer. J Natl Cancer Inst 96:621–628
de Azambuja E, Cardoso F, de Castro G, Jr., Colozza M, Mano MS, Durbecq V, Sotiriou C, Larsimont D, Piccart-Gebhart MJ, Paesmans M (2007) Ki-67 as prognostic marker in early breast cancer: a meta-analysis of published studies involving 12,155 patients. Br J Cancer 96:1504–1513
Demark-Wahnefried W, Polascik TJ, George SL, Switzer BR, Madden JF, Ruffin MT, Snyder DC, Owzar K, Hars V, Albala DM, Walther PJ, Robertson CN, Moul JW, Dunn BK, Brenner D, Minasian L, Stella P, Vollmer RT (2008) Flaxseed supplementation (not dietary fat restriction) reduces prostate cancer proliferation rates in men presurgery. Cancer Epidemiol Biomarkers Prev 17:3577–3587
Drazen JM (2005) COX-2 inhibitors–a lesson in unexpected problems. N Engl J Med 352:1131–1132
Dunn BK, Richmond E, Ryan A, Ford LG (2010) A nutrient approach to prostate cancer prevention: the Selenium and Vitamin E Cancer Prevention Trial (SELECT). Nutr Cancer (in press)
Eng-Wong J, Zujewski JA (2004) Raloxifene and its role in breast cancer prevention. Expert Rev Anticancer Ther 4:523–532
Eng-Wong J, Orzano-Birgani J, Chow CK, Venzon D, Yao J, Galbo CE, Zujewski JA, Prindiville S (2008) Effect of raloxifene on mammographic density and breast magnetic resonance imaging in premenopausal women at increased risk for breast cancer. Cancer Epidemiol Biomarkers Prev 17:1696–1701
Fabian CJ, Kimler BF (2006) Mammographic density: use in risk assessment and as a biomarker in prevention trials. J Nutr 136:2705S–2708S

Fabian CJ, Kimler BF (2007) Use of biomarkers for breast cancer risk assessment and prevention. J Steroid Biochem Mol Biol 106:31–39

Fabian CJ, Kimler BF, Brady DA, Mayo MS, Chang CH, Ferraro JA, Zalles CM, Stanton AL, Masood S, Grizzle WE, Boyd NF, Arneson DW, Johnson KA (2002) A phase II breast cancer chemoprevention trial of oral alpha-difluoromethylornithine: breast tissue, imaging, and serum and urine biomarkers. Clin Cancer Res 8:3105–3117

Fabian CJ, Kimler BF, Anderson J, Tawfik OW, Mayo MS, Burak WE Jr, O'Shaughnessy JA, Albain KS, Hyams DM, Budd GT, Ganz PA, Sauter ER, Beenken SW, Grizzle WE, Fruehauf JP, Arneson DW, Bacus JW, Lagios MD, Johnson KA, Browne D (2004) Breast cancer chemoprevention phase I evaluation of biomarker modulation by arzoxifene, a third generation selective estrogen receptor modulator. Clin Cancer Res 10:5403–5417

Fabian CJ, Kimler BF, Mayo MS, Khan SA (2005) Breast-tissue sampling for risk assessment and prevention. Endocr Relat Cancer 12:185–213

Fackler MJ, McVeigh M, Mehrotra J, Blum MA, Lange J, Lapides A, Garrett E, Argani P, Sukumar S (2004) Quantitative multiplex methylation-specific PCR assay for the detection of promoter hypermethylation in multiple genes in breast cancer. Cancer Res 64:4442–4452

Farmer H, McCabe N, Lord CJ, Tutt AN, Johnson DA, Richardson TB, Santarosa M, Dillon KJ, Hickson I, Knights C, Martin NM, Jackson SP, Smith GC, Ashworth A (2005) Targeting the DNA repair defect in BRCA mutant cells as a therapeutic strategy. Nature 434:917–921

Fisher B, Costantino JP, Wickerham DL, Redmond CK, Kavanah M, Cronin WM, Vogel V, Robidoux A, Dimitrov N, Atkins J, Daly M, Wieand S, Tan-Chiu E, Ford L, Wolmark N (1998) Tamoxifen for prevention of breast cancer: report of the National Surgical Adjuvant Breast and Bowel Project P-1 Study. J Natl Cancer Inst 90:1371–1388

Fisher B, Costantino JP, Wickerham DL, Cecchini RS, Cronin WM, Robidoux A, Bevers TB, Kavanah MT, Atkins JN, Margolese RG, Runowicz CD, James JM, Ford LG, Wolmark N (2005) Tamoxifen for the prevention of breast cancer: current status of the National Surgical Adjuvant Breast and Bowel Project P-1 study. J Natl Cancer Inst 97:1652–1662

Fleming TR (2005) Surrogate endpoints and FDA's accelerated approval process. Health Aff (Millwood) 24:67–78

Fleming TR, DeMets DL (1996) Surrogate end points in clinical trials: are we being misled? Ann Intern Med 125:605–613

Fong PC, Boss DS, Yap TA, Tutt A, Wu P, Mergui-Roelvink M, Mortimer P, Swaisland H, Lau A, O'Connor MJ, Ashworth A, Carmichael J, Kaye SB, Schellens JH, de Bono JS (2009) Inhibition of poly(ADP-ribose) polymerase in tumors from BRCA mutation carriers. N Engl J Med 361:123–134

Frank DH, Kimler BF, Fabian CJ, Ranger-Moore J, Yozwiak M, Bartels HG, Alberts DS, Bartels PH (2009) Digital image analysis of breast epithelial cells collected by random periareolar fine-needle aspirates (RPFNA) from women at high risk for breast cancer taking hormone replacement and the aromatase inhibitor, letrozole, for six months. Breast Cancer Res Treat 115:661–668

Freedman M, San MJ, O'Gorman J, Eckert S, Lippman ME, Lo SC, Walls EL, Zeng J (2001) Digitized mammography: a clinical trial of postmenopausal women randomly assigned to receive raloxifene, estrogen, or placebo. J Natl Cancer Inst 93:51–56

Gail MH, Brinton LA, Byar DP, Corle DK, Green SB, Schairer C, Mulvihill JJ (1989) Projecting individualized probabilities of developing breast cancer for white females who are being examined annually. J Natl Cancer Inst 81:1879–1886

Gohagan JK, Prorok PC, Hayes RB, Kramer BS (2000) The Prostate, Lung, Colorectal and Ovarian (PLCO) Cancer Screening Trial of the National Cancer Institute: history, organization, and status. Control Clin Trials 21:251S–272S

Goss PE, Richardson H, Chlebowski R, Johnston D, Sarto GE, Maunsell E, Ingle JN, Ales-Martinez JE (2007) National Cancer Institute of Canada Clinical Trials Group MAP.3 Trial: evaluation of exemestane to prevent breast cancer in postmenopausal women. Clin Breast Cancer 7:895–900

Hatsukami DK, Rennard S, Jorenby D, Fiore M, Koopmeiners J, de Vos A, Horwith G, Pentel PR (2005) Safety and immunogenicity of a nicotine conjugate vaccine in current smokers. Clin Pharmacol Ther 78:456–467

Imperiale TF, Ransohoff DF, Itzkowitz SH, Turnbull BA, Ross ME (2004) Fecal DNA versus fecal occult blood for colorectal-cancer screening in an average-risk population. N Engl J Med 351:2704–2714

Itzkowitz SH (2009) Incremental advances in excremental cancer detection tests. J Natl Cancer Inst 101:1225–1227

Jones LP, Li M, Halama ED, Ma Y, Lubet R, Grubbs CJ, Deng CX, Rosen EM, Furth PA (2005) Promotion of mammary cancer development by tamoxifen in a mouse model of BRCA1-mutation-related breast cancer. Oncogene 24:3554–3562

Jonsson S, Varella-Garcia M, Miller YE, Wolf HJ, Byers T, Braudrick S, Kiatsimkul P, Lewis M, Kennedy TC, Keith RL, Bjornsson J, McWilliams A, Lam S, Hirsch FR, Franklin WA (2008) Chromosomal aneusomy in bronchial high-grade lesions is associated with invasive lung cancer. Am J Respir Crit Care Med 177:342–347

Kelloff GJ, Lippman SM, Dannenberg AJ, Sigman CC, Pearce HL, Reid BJ, Szabo E, Jordan VC, Spitz MR, Mills GB, Papadimitrakopoulou VA, Lotan R, Aggarwal BB, Bresalier RS, Kim J, Arun B, Lu KH, Thomas ME, Rhodes HE, Brewer MA, Follen M, Shin DM, Parnes HL, Siegfried JM, Evans AA, Blot WJ, Chow WH, Blount PL, Maley CC, Wang KK, Lam S, Lee JJ, Dubinett SM, Engstrom PF, Meyskens FL Jr, O'Shaughnessy J, Hawk ET, Levin B, Nelson WG, Hong WK (2006) Progress in chemoprevention drug development: the promise of molecular biomarkers for prevention of intraepithelial neoplasia and cancer–a plan to move forward. Clin Cancer Res 12:3661–3697

Kong G, Kim HT, Wu K, DeNardo D, Hilsenbeck SG, Xu XC, Lamph WW, Bissonnette R, Dannenberg AJ, Brown PH (2005) The retinoid X receptor-selective retinoid, LGD1069, down-regulates cyclooxygenase-2 expression in human breast cells through transcription factor crosstalk: implications for molecular-based chemoprevention. Cancer Res 65:3462–3469

Kramer BS, Hagerty KL, Justman S, Somerfield MR, Albertsen PC, Blot WJ, Ballentine CH, Costantino JP, Epstein JI, Godley PA, Harris RP, Wilt TJ, Wittes J, Zon R, Schellhammer P (2009) Use of 5-alpha-reductase inhibitors for prostate cancer chemoprevention: American Society of Clinical Oncology/American Urological Association 2008 Clinical Practice Guideline. J Clin Oncol 27: 1502–1516

Kumar AS, Benz CC, Shim V, Minami CA, Moore DH, Esserman LJ (2008) Estrogen receptor-negative breast cancer is less likely to arise among lipophilic statin users. Cancer Epidemiol Biomarkers Prev 17:1028–1033

Kumar-Sinha C, Tomlins SA, Chinnaiyan AM (2008) Recurrent gene fusions in prostate cancer. Nat Rev Cancer 8:497–511

Lam S, McWilliams A, LeRiche J, MacAulay C, Wattenberg L, Szabo E (2006) A phase I study of myo-inositol for lung cancer chemoprevention. Cancer Epidemiol Biomarkers Prev 15:1526–1531

Laxman B, Morris DS, Yu J, Siddiqui J, Cao J, Mehra R, Lonigro RJ, Tsodikov A, Wei JT, Tomlins SA, Chinnaiyan AM (2008) A first-generation multiplex biomarker analysis of urine for the early detection of prostate cancer. Cancer Res 68:645–649

Lewis CM, Cler LR, Bu DW, Zochbauer-Muller S, Milchgrub S, Naftalis EZ, Leitch AM, Minna JD, Euhus DM (2005) Promoter hypermethylation in benign breast epithelium in relation to predicted breast cancer risk. Clin Cancer Res 11:166–172

Li Y, Brown PH (2009) Prevention of ER-negative breast cancer. Recent Results Cancer Res 181: 121–134

Lippman SM, Klein EA, Goodman PJ, Lucia MS, Thompson IM, Ford LG, Parnes HL, Minasian LM, Gaziano JM, Hartline JA, Parsons JK, Bearden JD III, Crawford ED, Goodman GE, Claudio J, Winquist E, Cook ED, Karp DD, Walther P, Lieber MM, Kristal AR, Darke AK, Arnold KB, Ganz PA, Santella RM, Albanes D, Taylor PR, Probstfield JL, Jagpal TJ, Crowley JJ, Meyskens FL Jr, Baker LH, Coltman CA Jr (2009) Effect of selenium and vitamin E on risk of prostate cancer and other cancers: the Selenium and Vitamin E Cancer Prevention Trial (SELECT). JAMA 301:39–51

Lucia MS, Epstein JI, Goodman PJ, Darke AK, Reuter VE, Civantos F, Tangen CM, Parnes HL, Lippman SM, La Rosa FG, Kattan MW, Crawford ED, Ford LG, Coltman CA Jr, Thompson IM (2007) Finasteride and high-grade prostate cancer in the Prostate Cancer Prevention Trial. J Natl Cancer Inst 99:1375–1383

Mandrekar SJ, Sargent DJ (2009) Clinical trial designs for predictive biomarker validation: theoretical considerations and practical challenges. J Clin Oncol 27:4027–4034

Meyskens FL Jr, Gerner EW (1999) Development of difluoromethylornithine (DFMO) as a chemoprevention agent. Clin Cancer Res 5: 945–951

Meyskens FL Jr, McLaren CE, Pelot D, Fujikawa-Brooks S, Carpenter PM, Hawk E, Kelloff G, Lawson MJ, Kidao J, McCracken J, Albers CG, Ahnen DJ, Turgeon DK, Goldschmid S, Lance P, Hagedorn CH, Gillen DL, Gerner EW (2008) Difluoromethylornithine plus sulindac for the prevention of sporadic colorectal adenomas: a randomized placebo-controlled, double-blind trial. Cancer Prev Res 1:32–38

National Cancer Institute (2010) NIH State-of-the-Science Conference: Enhancing Use and Quality of Colorectal Cancer Screening. February 2–4, 2010, Bethesda, MD, 2010. http://consensus.nih.gov/2010/colorectalstatement.htm. Accessed February 26, 2010

Natrajan R, Weigelt B, Mackay A, Geyer FC, Grigoriadis A, Tan DS, Jones C, Lord CJ, Vatcheva R, Rodriguez-Pinilla SM, Palacios J, Ashworth A, Reis-Filho JS (2010) An integrative genomic and transcriptomic analysis reveals molecular pathways and networks regulated by copy number aberrations in basal-like, HER2 and luminal cancers. Breast Cancer Res Treat 121:575–89

NLST (2010) NLST: National Lung Screening Trial. National Cancer Institute, Jan 3, 2010. http://www.cancer.gov/nlst. Accessed February 26, 2010

Pepe MS, Etzioni R, Feng Z, Potter JD, Thompson ML, Thornquist M, Winget M, Yasui Y (2001) Phases of biomarker development for early detection of cancer. J Natl Cancer Inst 93:1054–1061

Pepe MS, Feng Z, Janes H, Bossuyt PM, Potter JD (2008) Pivotal evaluation of the accuracy of a biomarker used for classification or prediction: standards for study design. J Natl Cancer Inst 100:1432–1438

Polyak K (2009) Molecular markers for the diagnosis and management of ductal carcinoma in situ. NIH State-of-the-Science Conference: Diagnosis and Management of Ductal Carcinoma In Situ (DCIS). September 22–24, Bethesda, MD. NIH State-of-the-Science Conference: Diagnosis and Management of Ductal Carcinoma In Situ (DCIS), September 22–24, Bethesda, MD, 2009. http://consensus.nih.gov/2009/dcisstatement.htm. Accessed February 26, 2010

Qiu J, Choi G, Li L, Wang H, Pitteri SJ, Pereira-Faca SR, Krasnoselsky AL, Randolph TW, Omenn GS, Edelstein C, Barnett MJ, Thornquist MD, Goodman GE, Brenner DE, Feng Z, Hanash SM (2008) Occurrence of autoantibodies to annexin I, 14-3-3 theta and LAMR1 in prediagnostic lung cancer sera. J Clin Oncol 26:5060–5066

Ransohoff DF, Feinstein AR (1978) Problems of spectrum and bias in evaluating the efficacy of diagnostic tests. N Engl J Med 299:926–930

Ransohoff DF, Gourlay ML (2010) Sources of bias in specimens for research about molecular markers for cancer. J Clin Oncol 28:698–704

Ronnov-Jessen L, Bissell MJ (2009) Breast cancer by proxy: can the microenvironment be both the cause and consequence? Trends Mol Med 15:5–13

Sardana G, Dowell B, Diamandis EP (2008) Emerging biomarkers for the diagnosis and prognosis of prostate cancer. Clin Chem 54:1951–1960

Schatzkin A, Gail M (2002) The promise and peril of surrogate end points in cancer research. Nat Rev Cancer 2:19–27

Schatzkin A, Freedman LS, Schiffman MH, Dawsey SM (1990) Validation of intermediate end points in cancer research. J Natl Cancer Inst 82:1746–1752

Schroy PC III, Heeren TC (2005) Patient perceptions of stool-based DNA testing for colorectal cancer screening. Am J Prev Med 28:208–214

Sreekumar A, Poisson LM, Rajendiran TM, Khan AP, Cao Q, Yu J, Laxman B, Mehra R, Lonigro RJ, Li Y, Nyati MK, Ahsan A, Kalyana-Sundaram S, Han B, Cao X, Byun J, Omenn GS, Ghosh D, Pennathur S, Alexander DC, Berger A, Shuster JR, Wei JT, Varambally S, Beecher C, Chinnaiyan AM (2009) Metabolomic profiles delineate potential role for sarcosine in prostate cancer progression. Nature 457:910–914

Tan-Chiu E, Wang J, Costantino JP, Paik S, Butch C, Wickerham DL, Fisher B, Wolmark N (2003) Effects of tamoxifen on benign breast disease in women at high risk for breast cancer. J Natl Cancer Inst 95:302–307

Thompson IM, Goodman PJ, Tangen CM, Lucia MS, Miller GJ, Ford LG, Lieber MM, Cespedes RD, Atkins JN, Lippman SM, Carlin SM, Ryan A, Szczepanek CM, Crowley JJ, Coltman CA Jr (2003) The influence of finasteride on the development of prostate cancer. N Engl J Med 349:215–224

Thompson IM, Pauler DK, Goodman PJ, Tangen CM, Lucia MS, Parnes HL, Minasian LM, Ford LG, Lippman SM, Crawford ED, Crowley JJ, Coltman CA Jr (2004) Prevalence of prostate cancer among men with a prostate-specific antigen level < or =4.0 ng per milliliter. N Engl J Med 350:2239–2246

Tice JA, Cummings SR, Smith-Bindman R, Ichikawa L, Barlow WE, Kerlikowske K (2008) Using clinical factors and mammographic breast density to estimate breast cancer risk: development and validation of a new predictive model. Ann Intern Med 148:337–347

Tomlins SA, Rhodes DR, Perner S, Dhanasekaran SM, Mehra R, Sun XW, Varambally S, Cao X, Tchinda J, Kuefer R, Lee C, Montie JE, Shah RB, Pienta KJ, Rubin MA, Chinnaiyan AM (2005) Recurrent fusion of TMPRSS2 and ETS transcription factor genes in prostate cancer. Science 310:644–648

Tomlins SA, Rhodes DR, Yu J, Varambally S, Mehra R, Perner S, Demichelis F, Helgeson BE, Laxman B, Morris DS, Cao Q, Cao X, Andren O, Fall K, Johnson L, Wei JT, Shah RB, Al-Ahmadie H, Eastham JA, Eggener SE, Fine SW, Hotakainen K, Stenman UH, Tsodikov A, Gerald WL, Lilja H, Reuter VE, Kantoff PW, Scardino PT, Rubin MA, Bjartell AS, Chinnaiyan AM (2008) The role of SPINK1 in ETS rearrangement-negative prostate cancers. Cancer Cell 13:519–528

Vogel VG, Costantino JP, Wickerham DL, Cronin WM, Cecchini RS, Atkins JN, Bevers TB, Fehrenbacher L, Pajon ER, Wade JL 3rd, Robidoux A, Margolese RG, James J, Runowicz CD, Ganz PA, Reis SE, McCaskill-Stevens W, Ford LG, Jordan VC, Wolmark N. National Surgical Adjuvant Breast and Bowel Project (2010) Update of the National Surgical Adjuvant Breast and Bowel Project Study of Tamoxifen and Raloxifene (STAR) P-2 Trial: Preventing breast cancer. Cancer Prev Res 3:696–706.

Vourlekis JS, Szabo E (2004) Use of markers for the detection and treatment of lung cancer. Dis Markers 20:71–85

Wagner JA (2002) Overview of biomarkers and surrogate endpoints in drug development. Dis Markers 18:41–46

Wang W, Srivastava S (2010) Strategic approach to validating methylated genes as biomarkers for breast cancer. Cancer Prev Res (Phila Pa) 3:16–24

Yang WT, Lewis MT, Hess K, Wong H, Tsimelzon A, Karadag N, Cairo M, Wei C, Meric-Bernstam F, Brown P, Arun B, Hortobagyi GN, Sahin A, Chang JC (2010) Decreased TGFbeta signaling and increased COX2 expression in high risk women with increased mammographic breast density. Breast Cancer Res Treat 119:305–314

zur Hausen H (2000) Papillomaviruses causing cancer: evasion from host-cell control in early events in carcinogenesis. J Natl Cancer Inst 92:690-698

Targeting Polyamines and Inflammation for Cancer Prevention

4

Naveen Babbar and Eugene W. Gerner

Abstract Increased polyamine synthesis and inflammation have long been associated with intraepithelial neoplasia, which are risk factors for cancer development in humans. Targeting polyamine metabolism (by use of polyamine synthesis inhibitors or polyamine catabolism activators) and inflammation (by use of nonsteroidal anti-inflammatory drugs) has been studied for many cancers, including colon, prostate, and skin. Genetic epidemiology results indicate that a genetic variant associated with the expression of a polyamine biosynthetic gene is associated with risk of colon and prostate cancers. A clinical trial of difluoromethylornithine (DFMO), a selective inhibitor of polyamine synthesis, showed that the 1 year treatment duration reduced prostate volume and serum prostate-specific antigen doubling time in men with a family history of prostate cancer. A second, clinical trial of DFMO in combination with sulindac, a NSAID in patients with prior colon polyps found that the 3-year treatment was associated with a 70% reduction of all, and over a 90% reduction of advanced and/or multiple metachronous colon adenomas. In this chapter, we discuss that similar combination prevention strategies of targeting polyamines and inflammation can be effective in reducing risk factors associated with the development of human cancers.

N. Babbar
Research and Development, Osmetech Molecular Diagnostic, 757 S Raymond Avenue, Pasadena, CA 91105, USA
e-mail: naveen.babbar@osmetech.com

E.W. Gerner (✉)
Arizona Cancer Center, University of Arizona, 1515 North Campbell Avenue, Tucson, AZ 85724, USA
e-mail: egerner@azcc.arizona.edu

Abbreviations

APAO	FAD-dependent polyamine oxidase
DFMO	D,L-α-difluoromethylornithine
NSAID	Non-steroidal anti-inflammatory drug
ODC	Ornithine decarboxylase
SAMDC	S-adenosylmethionine Decarboxylase
SAT1	Spermidine/Spermine N^1-Acetyltransferase
APC	Adenomatous polyposis coli
SMO	Spermine oxidase
OAZ	Ornithine decarboxylase antizyme
NOS	Nitric oxide synthases
PPAR	Gamma: Peroxisomal proliferator activated receptor γ
COX-2	Cyclooxygenase-2
TNFalpha	Tumor necrosis factor-α
BCC	Basal cell carcinoma

H.-J. Senn and F. Otto (eds.), *Clinical Cancer Prevention*,
Recent Results in Cancer Research 188, DOI: 10.1007/978-3-642-10858-7_4,

4

FAP	Familial adenomatous polyposis
PIA	Proliferative inflammatory atrophy
PIN	Prostatic intraepithelial neoplasia
PSA	Prostate specific antigen
NMSC	Nonmelanoma skin cancers
SCC	Squamous cell carcinoma

4.1 Introduction

Inflammation plays an essential role in the initiation and progression of many types of human epithelial cancers. Chronic inflammation leads to activation of macrophages and other inflammatory cells that generate increased amounts of growth factors and cytokines, as well as reactive oxygen and nitrogen species that may cause DNA damage. Persistent activation of macrophages can lead to continuous tissue damage in a microenvironment that sustains proliferation of damaged cells, thus predisposing areas of chronic inflammation to neoplasia. Polyamines are aliphatic cations present in all cells, whose levels are intricately controlled by their transport and metabolic enzymes. Polyamines are essential for cell growth and proliferation, and have also been shown to play an important role in inflammation-induced carcinogenesis. Cells have developed complex regulatory machinery to finely control intracellular polyamine pools, as dysregulation of polyamine metabolism can have serious effects on cell growth. Increased polyamine synthesis has been detected as a product of inflammation, and elevated intracellular polyamine pools are frequently observed in actively proliferating cells, including tumor cells. This review will highlight the studies and research which is being done in targeting either inflammation or polyamines for the prevention of cancers. Further, we will provide rationale for designing clinical trials which should target both inflammation and polyamines for the increased chem.-preventive actions.

4.2 Polyamines, Inflammation, and Cancer

4.2.1 Polyamine Metabolism

Polyamines (putrescine, spermidine and spermine) are aliphatic polycations present in all cells. They have pleiotropic effects on cell physiology and play a relevant role in cell proliferation (Thomas and Thomas 2001). Cells have developed complex regulatory machinery, which controls intracellular polyamine pool sizes in a fast and accurate manner by the combined action of de novo synthesis, uptake, catabolism, and uptake of polyamines. The regulatory machinery consists of finely regulated enzymatic steps. These include reactions catalyzed by the biosynthetic enzymes, ornithine decarboxylase (ODC), S-adenosylmethionine decarboxylase (SAMDC), and the spermidine and spermine synthases. Polyamine catabolism is catalyzed by the combined actions of spermidine/spermine N^1-acetyltransferase (SAT1) and the FAD-dependent polyamine oxidase (APAO) or directly by spermine oxidase (SMO). Intracellular levels of polyamines are tightly controlled. The key enzymes involved in both metabolic pathways, in particular ODC, SAMDC, SAT1, and SMO, are present in low abundance, exhibit rapid turnover, and are under complex transcriptional and posttranscriptional regulation. As their half-lives are very short (Coleman et al. 1994), their expression levels can change by several orders of magnitude very quickly in response to different types of stimuli. ODC is typically induced by growth-promoting factors. It has been shown to be critical in cell transformation, and thus has been suggested to be a proto-oncogene. It undergoes complex regulation, mostly based on the induction of a unique, nonenzymatic, regulatory protein named ornithine decarboxylase antizyme (OAZ) (Hayashi et al. 1996).

Polyamine catabolism occurs through two distinct pathways, and uses a total of three enzymes: spermidine/spermine N^1-acetyltransferase (SAT1), acetyl polyamine oxidase (APAO), and spermine oxidase (SMO). SAT1 acetylates both spermine and spermidine, thus providing acetylated polyamines as substrates for further back-conversion to spermidine or putrescine by APAO. Alternatively, spermine can be directly oxidized back to spermidine through SMO. Importantly, the oxidization reactions of both APAO and SMO result in the generation of the toxic byproduct, hydrogen peroxide (H_2O_2). This H_2O_2, a reactive oxygen species (ROS), has been shown to play an essential role in the DNA damage-associated changes observed following elevated levels of polyamine catabolism (Fig. 4.1). Furthermore, the depletion of intracellular polyamine pools that typically accompanies induction of polyamine catabolism can itself be growth inhibitory (Seiler 1987).

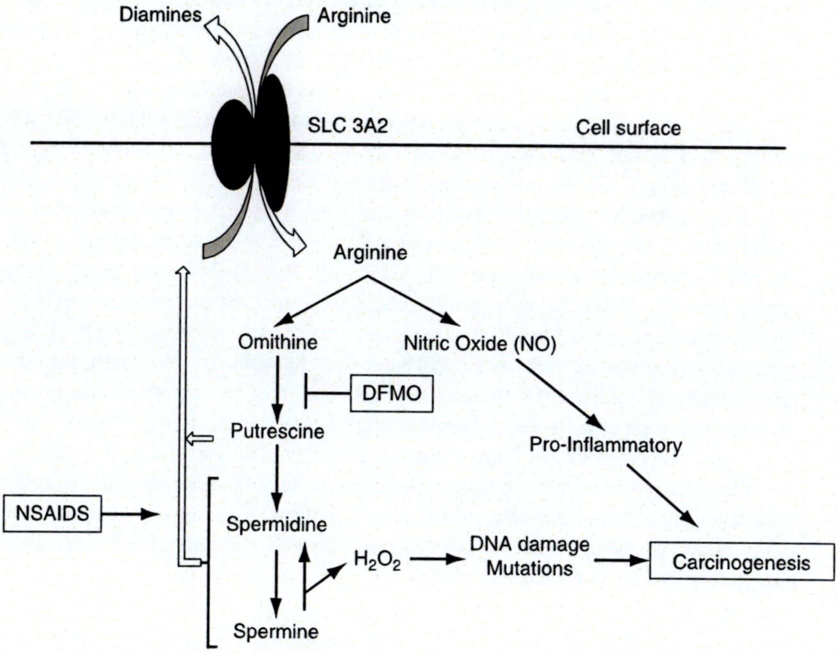

Fig. 4.1 Polyamine Metabolism, Inflammation and Carcinogenesis. The processes of polyamine metabolism and inflammation are coupled, in part, by the solute carrier transporter SLC3A2, which imports the amino acid arginine using diamines as the antiport molecule (Uemura et al. 2008). SLC3A2 is physically associated with the spermidine/spermine N[1]-acetyltransferase (SAT1), which acetylates spermidine and spermine and target them for export by this transporter. As shown in this figure, the activity of the surface transporter to import arginine can be enhanced by increasing polyamine synthesis and/or export, as occurs in human prostate carcinogenesis (Bettuzzi et al. 2000). Inhibition of polyamine synthesis, by agents such as DFMO and activation of polyamine catabolism and export by drugs such as the NSAIDS, reduce cell and tissue polyamines and subsequently arginine transport. The consequence of arginine pool size reduction is to reduce the levels of the pro-inflammatory molecule NO. Reduced NO, along with reduced polyamines, is associated with reduced carcinogenesis. Spermine can be oxidized to spermidine with the generation of H_2O_2 in the process, which can in turn lead to DNA damage which is pro-carcinogenic (Babbar and Casero 2006). Increased catabolism/export by NSAIDs leads to a decrease in spermine, thereby leading to decreased production of the DNA damaging H_2O_2

4.2.2 Polyamines and Cancer

For more than 25 years, it has been recognized that there is a strong association between high levels of polyamines and rapid proliferation (Russell and Snyder, 1968). In both rodent and human neoplastic cells and tissues, polyamine contents are often elevated when compared to normal cells and tissues. Polyamine metabolism is an integral component of the mechanism of carcinogenesis in epithelial tissues. Increases in ODC are often associated with initiation of normal cell growth and sustained neoplastic cell growth.

Cancer development is a multistep process, during which genetic alterations confer specific growth advantages, thereby driving the progressive transformation from normal cells to malignant cancer cells. Malignant growth is characterized by several key changes: self-sufficiency of growth signals, insensitivity to antigrowth signals, escape from apoptosis, unregulated proliferation potential, enhanced angiogenesis, and metastasis (Hanahan and Weinberg 2000). Each of these shifts is complicated and accomplished by the combined efforts of various signaling processes. Inflammation is a physiologic response to tissue damage resulting from microbial pathogen infection, chemical irritation, and/or wounding. However, if inflammation resolution is dysregulated, the cellular response changes to a pattern of chronic inflammation, in which the inflammatory foci are dominated by macrophages and other inflammatory cells that generate even greater amounts of growth factors and cytokines, as well as reactive oxygen and nitrogen species that may cause DNA damage. Persistent activation of macrophages can lead to continuous tissue damage (Macarthur et al. 2004) in a microenvironment that sustains proliferation of damaged cells, thus predisposing areas of chronic inflammation to neoplasia (Balkwill and Mantovani 2001).

The association between inflammation and cancer has been illustrated by numerous epidemiologic and clinical studies (Balkwill and Mantovani 2001; Coussens and Werb 2002). Causes of inflammation that have been linked to cancer include bacterial and viral infection (*Helicobacter pylori* for gastric adenocarcinoma (Coussens and Werb 2002; Macarthur et al. 2004), *hepatitis B and C* for hepatocellular carcinoma (Block et al. 2003), and *human papillomavirus* for penile cancers), or noninfective physical and/or chemical irritants. The risk of developing esophageal, pancreatic, and gallbladder cancers may be increased by certain inflammatory diseases, such as esophagitis, Barrett's metaplasia, and chronic pancreatitis (Macarthur et al. 2004; Whitcomb 2004). Possible associations have also been described between Marjolin's ulcer and skin carcinoma (Macarthur et al. 2004); asbestos and mesothelioma (Macarthur et al. 2004); silica, cigarette smoke, and bronchial cancer (Macarthur et al. 2004); chronic asthma and lung cancer (Vesterinen et al. 1993); and pelvic inflammatory disease or ovarian epithelial inflammation and ovarian cancer (Risch and Howe 1995; Macarthur et al. 2004).

Polyamines have been shown to play an important role in inflammation-induced carcinogenesis (Russell and Snyder 1968). Increased polyamine synthesis has been detected as a product of inflammation, and elevated intracellular polyamine pools are frequently observed in actively proliferating cells, including tumor cells. In one study, parasitic infection of the small intestine led to increased mucosal hyperplasia with elevated polyamine biosynthesis (Wang et al. 1991). Additionally, *H. pylori* infection has been demonstrated to increase expression and activity of polyamine biosynthetic enzymes (Gobert et al. 2002). Meanwhile, intracellular levels of the polyamines themselves are capable of affecting inflammation. The polyamine spermine has been shown to inhibit pro-inflammatory cytokine synthesis in human mononuclear cells (Zhang et al. 1997), as well as nitric oxide-mediated intestinal damage (ter Steege et al. 1999).

Polyamine and nitric oxide metabolism are linked by their common dependence on arginine, which is the substrate for nitric oxide synthases

(NOS) and arginase. NOSs produce nitric oxide and arginases produce ornithine, the substrate for putrescine biosynthesis. One member of a di- and acetyl-polyamine exporter was recently shown to be the solute carrier family member SLC3A2 (Uemura et al. 2008). SLC3A2 was found to export di- and acetyl-polyamines via a mechanism involving arginine antiport. Deletion of NOS2 alleles in genetically engineered mouse models of inflammation and intestinal carcinogenesis suppress both these processes (Yerushalmi et al. 2006; Bernstein et al. 2007). Pharmacological depletion of tissue polyamine contents likewise suppresses arginine-dependent colonic carcinogenesis in *Apc*$^{Min/+}$ mice (Yerushalmi et al. 2006b). Thus, polyamines, acting via SLC3A2, might be an important component in the transport of arginine for the production of pro-inflammatory molecule nitric oxide (Fig. 4.1).

4.3 Roles of Inflammation and Polyamines in Prostate Cancer

4.3.1 Polyamines and Prostate Cancer

The prostate and prostatic secretions have played an important role in our current understanding of polyamines. The prostate has one of the highest polyamine concentrations of any tissue. The initial identification of one of the polyamines, i.e. spermine, was reported in human semen as early as the seventeenth century by Antonie van Leeuwenhoek. In rat prostate, spermidine is the predominant polyamine, whereas in the human prostate spermine is present in high amounts. The activities of the polyamine biosynthetic enzymes ODC, SAMDC, and spermidine synthase are induced by androgens in a coordinated way, and expression of these enzymes is primarily localized to the glandular epithelial cells of the prostate (Fjosne et al. 1992; Cyriac et al. 2002). Studies on the murine ODC gene revealed that the ODC promoter contains an androgen-responsive element-like sequence that can bind to the androgen receptor in vitro (Crozat et al. 1992). Studies on the rat and human prostate-derived tumors showed that ODC activity was substantially higher in the more malignant sublines (Schipper et al. 2000). Immunoblot analysis of tissue specimens of patients with prostate cancer showed a significantly elevated protein expression of ODC in the cancerous tissues as compared with the benign tissues (Mohan et al. 1999). Moreover, studies on the expression levels of the ODC gene in a series of 23 human prostate cancers dissected from radical prostatectomy specimens revealed significantly increased ODC expression.

4.3.2 Polyamines, Inflammation, and Prostate Cancer

In the prostate, studies suggest widespread asymptomatic prostatitis arising from a multitude of stimuli, including microbial infection and dietary components. Emerging epidemiological, histopathological, and molecular evidence suggests that such inflammation may be associated with the development of putatively preneoplastic proliferative inflammatory atrophy (PIA), as well as prostatic intraepithelial neoplasia (PIN) and prostate cancer. The most compelling molecular evidence for a mechanistic association between inflammation and prostate cancer is the appearance of somatic epigenetic alterations of certain androgen-regulated differentiation genes and candidate oncogenes in preneoplastic PIA lesions that are reminiscent of those known to be present in prostate cancers (Bardia et al. 2009). Further PIA lesions consist of regions of atrophic epithelium exhibiting an elevated proportion of proliferating cells, association with inflammatory cells, and increased expression of the pro-inflammatory enzyme cyclooxygenase-2 (COX-2) (De Marzo et al. 2007a). In addition, various inflammatory stimuli, including sexually transmitted infections, dietary factors, exposure to estrogen, and urine reflux, have been implicated as potential environmental triggers of prostatic inflammation (De Marzo et al. 2007b). Even though the precise molecular mechanisms linking the inflammatory microenvironment to potentially carcinogenic events including DNA damage, tumor suppressor gene inactivation, and increased proliferation remain to be identified, until recently it was shown that PINs have an increased expression of SMO. SMO is induced in human gastric and lung epithelial cells by *H. pylori* infection and the pro-inflammatory cytokine tumor necrosis factor-a (TNF-a), respectively, and this increase in SMO activity produces sufficient H_2O_2 to cause oxidative DNA damage and apoptosis (Xu et al. 2004; Babbar and Casero 2006). This increased expression of SMO suggested the role SMO plays in the development of precursor PIN lesions and initiation events in prostate carcinogenesis (Goodwin et al. 2008) as it is known that in certain epithelial cells, increased SMO expression produces sufficient H_2O_2 to cause oxidative DNA damage and apoptosis (Xu et al. 2004; Babbar and Casero 2006).

4.3.3 Targeting Polyamines and Inflammation in Prostate Cancer

D,L-α-difluoromethylornithine (DFMO), the most widely studied inhibitor of ODC, has striking inhibitory effects on the growth of cultured prostatic cancer cells. Numerous in vitro and in vivo studies with DFMO in prostate models have shown its efficacy in decreasing prostate polyamine levels, tumor growth, prostate growth, and regrowth. DFMO-inhibited growth of PC-3, PC-82, and androgen-stimulated LNCaP cells could be reversed by exogenously added polyamines or their acetylated derivatives. Rodents were castrated with subsequent decrease in prostate size and polyamine content. With the return of exogenous androgens, the prostatic atrophy was readily reversed and polyamine content was normalized. DFMO markedly slowed prostatic weight gain from the androgens to half of the weight of the controls and blocked increases in putrescine and spermidine levels in the prostate (Danzin et al. 1979). Inhibition of polyamine synthesis by 1% DFMO showed marked reduction in weight and volume of the prostate as well as metastasis (Gupta et al. 2000), while activation of polyamine catabolism by over-expression of SAT1 in the transgenic adenocarcinoma mouse prostate model had smaller weights of their prostates at 30 and 36 weeks and better histologic scores (Kee et al. 2004). In humans, a prostate study also showed no risk stratification for cancer based on the ODC polymorphism alone, but those with an A allele when linked with androgen receptor polymorphisms (CAG repeats <22) had an odds ratio of 2 for prostate cancer. Smoking has also been linked to prostate cancer risk in men with an A allele only (Visvanathan et al. 2004). A prospective, randomized double-blind, placebo-controlled clinical trial of DFMO showed that the 1-year treatment duration reduced putrescine levels, prostate volume, and serum prostate-specific antigen (PSA) doubling time in men with a family history of prostate cancer (Simoneau et al. 2008). In addition, stratification by ODC genotype showed that men with the AA or AG genotype showed a reduction in putrescine level and decrease in total prostate volume, but no reduction in these variables were seen in men with the GG genotype. A promising alternative to the use of inhibitors of polyamine biosynthetic enzymes is the application of synthetic polyamine analogs such as BENSpm, DENSpm, BE-4-4-4-4, etc. which function by activating the polyamine catabolism. Multiple studies showed that these analogs have differential effects on cell growth and polyamine homeostasis in different prostatic carcinoma cells, i.e. the androgen-independent DU-145 cells were the most sensitive, whereas the well-differentiated androgen-dependent LNCaP cells were relatively insensitive. Treatment with these analogs evoked intracellular accumulation of the analog and various regulatory responses, for example, down-regulation of polyamine biosynthesis, the induction of the catabolic enzyme spermidine/spermine-N1-acetyltransferase (SAT1), and the depletion or decrease of the natural polyamines.

NSAIDs, as nonsteroidal anti-inflammatory drugs, have been extensively studied in relation to its chemopreventive actions in prostate cancer. Numerous preclinical studies using selective and nonselective COX inhibitors for prostate cancer prevention and treatment have been shown to promote inactivation of Bcl-2, inactivation of Akt, reduction of NF-kappaB p65, down-regulation of androgen receptor activity, up-regulation of the p75 NTR tumor suppressor, and increase in detoxification enzyme GSTP1, all of which could contribute to potential tumor inhibitory effects. Population-based studies of aspirin intake have hinted at a protective effect on prostate cancer risk (Jacobs et al. 2005; Mahmud et al. 2006). The inverse association between aspirin use and prostate cancer appears stronger for higher frequency use, for greater duration of use, among younger men, and for advanced prostate cancer. The association between nonaspirin NSAIDs and prostate cancer in population studies is more varied. The systematic review by Mahmud et al. found that nonaspirin NSAIDs were inversely associated with prostate cancer (OR = 0.87, 95% CI: 0.61, 1.23), although this finding was not statistically significant ($P = 0.43$), and substantial heterogeneity was evident between studies ($P = 0.005$). One major unresolved issue that might add clarity to the population studies concerns the fraction of ingested aspirin or of the different nonaspirin NSAIDs appearing in prostate tissues and/or the lumens of prostate glands (the location of many of the inflammatory cells). Careful pharmacological studies, using drugs like aspirin and desipramine as model agents, have suggested that factors such as hydrophobicity, pH–pKa partitioning, and metabolism, might affect the propensity of drugs to pass into the prostate and seminal vesicles. For protection against prostatic carcinogenesis, drugs that are incapable of accumulating in the prostate at sufficient concentrations to attenuate inflammation are unlikely to be of great benefit.

While there have been clinical trials evaluating the combined effects of polyamine modulators (DFMO) with aspirin or other nonaspirin NSAIDs on colorectal cancer incidence, there has been no randomized clinical trial testing the effect of aspirin in combination with polyamine modulators on prostate cancer incidence. When considered together, the basic, preclinical, epidemiological, and limited clinical trial evidence supports further study of the protective effects of aspirin and/or nonaspirin NSAIDs with DFMO against prostate cancer development. Identifying a subpopulation of patients that are most likely to respond to NSAIDs or DFMO, based on biomarker profile, and utilizing NSAIDs as targeted therapies are most likely to optimize success.

4.4 Roles of Inflammation and Polyamines in Colon Cancer

4.4.1 Polyamines and Colon Cancer

Colon carcinogenesis involves several intermediate stages. Normal colonic epithelium gives rise to small adenomas and then to large adenomas, which subsequently progress to metastatic carcinomas (Fearon and Vogelstein 1990). In colon cancer tissue, the activities of polyamine-synthesizing enzymes and polyamine content are increased 10- to 15-fold in comparison to normal colonic epithelium (Elitsur et al. 1992), and polyamines have therefore been considered even as specific markers for neoplastic proliferation in the colon (Higuchi and Wang 1995). ODC activity and expression have been among the first biomarkers of neoplastic proliferation: as early as 1984 it was shown that ODC activity correlates with risk for neoplastic transformation in patients with colonic adenomatous polyposis (Luk and Baylin 1984). ODC activity correlates also with a degree of dysplasia in Barrett's esophagus (Gerner et al. 1994) and different stages of colonic carcinogenesis (Giardiello et al. 1997). Two of the most commonly mutated genes in colon cancer found in this study include the adenomatous polyposis coli (APC) tumor suppressor gene and the K-RAS oncogene, both of which have been shown to regulate the expression of several polyamine metabolic genes (Erdman et al. 1999; Ignatenko et al. 2004). Polyamine synthesis and levels of individual polyamines increase in colorectal cancers, compared to adjacent apparently normal mucosal tissue (Hixson et al. 1993). One mechanism by which APC mutations promote tumorigenesis is to increase transcription of ODC, via a c-MYC dependent process, and polyamine synthesis in human cells and $Apc^{Min/+}$ mice (Erdman et al. 1999; Fultz and Gerner 2002). ODC enzyme activity and polyamine contents are also elevated in the apparently normal colonic mucosa of presymptomatic, genotype-positive individuals with familial adenomatous polyposis (FAP), an inherited syndrome caused by mutations/deletions in the APC gene. K-RAS acts to increase cell and tissue polyamine contents by increasing ODC enzyme activity and by own-regulating expression of the SAT1 via a transcriptional mechanism involving the peroxisomal proliferator activated receptor g (PPARg) (Ignatenko et al. 2004). Inactivation of PAO has been shown to impede colon carcinogenesis in dimethylhydrazine treated rat model (Halline and Brasitus 1990). Derivatives of spermidine and spermine, acetylated at the N^1 position by SAT1, have been shown to accumulate in neoplastic but not normal tissues during carcinogenesis in the rat model and in human cancer (Loser et al. 1990), probably reflecting high levels of these amines in neoplasia.

4.4.2 Polyamines, Inflammation, and Colon Cancer

Colonic bacteria provide sources of potential tumor-promoting polyamines and other luminal risk factors for colon cancer. These bacteria metabolize primary bile acids to secondary bile acids, which have been associated with colon cancers in humans and are capable of promoting colon carcinogenesis in rodent models. There have been multiple studies suggest a linkage between polyamines and inflammation, and polyamines, inflammation, and colon cancer (Bernstein et al. 2006, 2007; Yerushalmi et al. 2007a). This linkage may be more than simply an association. Microarray analysis of human colon cancer-derived cells identified SAT1 as a target of the nonsteroidal anti-inflammatory drug sulindac (Babbar et al. 2003). Sulindac and other nonsteroidal anti-inflammatory drug act by distinct transcriptional mechanisms to induce SAT1 and promote the export of diamines and acetylpolyamines in both human cell and mouse models (Babbar et al. 2006; Ignatenko et al. 2006). Polyamines are oxidized by several amine oxidases to produce reactive oxygen species and aldehydes (Babbar et al. 2007). Polyamines can also influence the expression of the pro-inflammatory gene cyclooxygenase 2 by a posttranscriptional mechanism (Parker and Gerner 2002).

4.4.3 Targeting Polyamines and Inflammation in Colon Cancer

NSAIDs have been used to treat arthritis since 1899, when the analgesic and anti-inflammatory effects of aspirin were first recognized. NSAIDs have been shown experimentally to stimulate apoptosis and to inhibit angiogenesis, two mechanisms that help to suppress malignant transformation and tumor growth. Numerous epidemiologic studies have found that long-term users of aspirin or other NSAIDs have a lower risk of colorectal adenomatous polyps and colorectal cancer than nonusers (Thun et al. 1991; Deutsch 1992; Paganini-Hill et al. 1992; Schreinemachers and Everson 1994; Goldberg 1996). Randomized clinical trials have confirmed that the NSAIDs, Sulindac (Giardiello et al. 1993; Stoner et al. 1999) and the selective COX-2 inhibitor celecoxib (Steinbach et al. 2000), effectively inhibit the growth of adenomatous polyps and cause regression of existing polyps in patients with FAP. Observations from our own studies and those of others indicate that several NSAIDs, which have the ability to suppress carcinogenesis in some tissues, activate SAT1 as part of their anticancer activity. These activation mechanisms are NSAID-specific (Babbar et al. 2006), but involve PPAR-gamma in the case of sulindac (Babbar et al. 2003).

Inhibitors of polyamine synthesis, such as DFMO, suppress intestinal and colon carcinogenesis in experimental murine models (Gerner et al. 2003). Further, there is evidence suggesting that diet and genetic host factors may distinguish between individuals who will and will not benefit from specific, high-priority colon cancer-preventive agents. Specifically, we have found that DFMO suppresses only the development of high-grade colon adenomas that form in the *Apc*$^{Min/+}$ mouse as a consequence of dietary supplementation of arginine at levels corresponding to arginine consumption in humans (Yerushalmi et al. 2007b). These results showed that the major effect of DFMO was to reduce the number of high risk, as determined by pathological high grade, adenomas while having little effect on the number of total colon adenomas.

Due to the suppressive effects of both NSAIDs and polyamine inhibitors on colon carcinogenesis, it was logical to assume that combination of these types of agents might lead to increased anticarcinogenic results. Further, combinations of these drugs could offer the potential of efficacy at much lower concentrations than would have required if they were used independently. Actually, evidence for the efficacy of targeting inflammation and polyamine synthesis for cancer chemoprevention began to accumulate over 20 years ago with the work of Nigro and colleagues (Nigro et al. 1986), which proposed the strategy of combination chemoprevention following the success of combination chemotherapy for certain types of cancer. Combination chemoprevention offered the prospect of reduced toxicities by lowering doses of individual agents. Many experimental studies have shown that DFMO acts at least additively with a number of NSAIDS, including the COX1 selective agent aspirin (Li et al. 1999), the COX2 selective agent celecoxib, and nonselective inhibitors of both COX1 and COX2, including piroxicam and sulindac (Lawson et al. 2000). Clinical evidence for beneficial effects of many NSAIDs on colon polyp formation has also accumulated – sulindac in high-risk individuals such as those with FAP (Giardiello et al. 1993), aspirin, and colon adenomas (Greenberg et al. 1993; Sandler et al. 2003). We have described that aspirin is able to decrease the risk of colon adenoma recurrence in a statistically significant manner, especially in individuals who were found to have a single nucleotide polymorphism (SNP) in the ODC promoter (Martinez et al. 2003). The relationship between this ODC SNP and aspirin and risk of polyp recurrence has now been independently corroborated in participants of a prospective randomized trial of aspirin for colon polyp prevention (Barry et al. 2006; Hubner et al. 2008). It is speculated that the mechanism of this association involves the combined action of the ODC-A allele-specific suppression of ODC transcription, and aspirin activation of SAT1 and polyamine export.

4

Meyskens et al. recently showed the dramatic efficacy of a combination of DFMO and the sulindac in a randomized double-blind, placebo-controlled phase III trial for colorectal adenoma prevention (Meyskens et al. 2008). This combination was markedly more effective in preventing metachronous colorectal adenomas when compared to other interventions, as highlighted in Table 4.1. In the Meyskens' trial, patients with a genetic risk of colon cancer or with current or prior colon or other cancers were excluded. Participants received the combination of DFMO (two 250-mg pills daily) and sulindac (one 150 mg pill daily), or placebo pills, for 3 years. Sulindac was used at a relatively low concentration to avoid any adverse cardiovascular (CV) events, which have been shown to occur in several randomized trials with cyclooxygenase-2-selective NSAIDs (Bertagnolli et al. 2006; Solomon et al. 2006) and assumed to occur with COX-2 nonselective NSAIDs including sulindac. The primary end points included adenoma recurrence and toxicity assessment. Treatment with DFMO and sulindac produced a 70% reduction in total polyps, and 91.5% reduction in both advanced adenomas and in patients with multiple recurrent adenomas, at the end of 3 years. Treatment-associated toxicities were rare but the risk of adverse CV event associated with DFMO/sulindac increased with a high, but not with a low, baseline CV risk score (Zell et al. 2009). These findings were consistent with data from larger studies, but due to small numbers, the study did not have sufficient power to study the statistical interaction between baseline CV risk and the intervention. This combination clinical trial of DFMO and sulindac provides as an important proof of principle that targeting polyamine metabolism and inflammation can be an effective strategy for reducing risk factors, such as colon adenomas, that are closely associated with the development of colon cancers in humans. This

Table 4.1 Comparison of recent colorectal polyp prevention trails.This table summarizes studies reported over the past decade that have evaluated a number of interventions for their potential to reduce metachronous colorectal polyps. These trials all accrued similar patient populations (i.e. patients with prior sporadic colorectal polyps) and employed similar intervention intervals (approximately 3 years in all cases). The numbers of patients in each trial were different and give an indication of the ability to detect differences between treatment and placebo groups. The metachronous adenoma rate in the placebo arms of these trials is listed, to show that the populations were similar in this regard

Intervention	Investigator (year)	Participants	Metachronous adenoma rate (%)	Intervention effect (relative risk or fraction placebo)
Calcium	(Baron et al. 1999)	832	38	0.85 ($P=0.03$)
Fiber	(Alberts et al. 2000)	1303	51	0.88 ($P=0.28$)
High Vegetable & Fruit/Low Fat	(Schatzkin et al. 2000)	1905	40	1.00
Aspirin	(Baron et al. 2003)	1084	47	0.81 (any) 0.59 (advanced)
Celebrex	(Bertagnolli et al. 2006)	2035	61 (any) 17 (advanced)	0.67 ($P<0.001$) 0.55 ($P<0.001$)
Celebrex	(Arber et al. 2006)	1561	49 (any) 10 (advanced)	0.64 ($P<0.001$) 0.49 ($P<0.001$)
Vioxx	(Baron et al. 2006)	2587	55	0.76 ($P<0.01$)
DFMO+Sulindac	(Meyskens et al. 2008)	375	42 (any) 11 (advanced)	0.31 ($P<0.001$) 0.08 ($P<0.001$)

strategy may be applicable for reduction of risk factors in other human cancers such as breast, lung, and prostate.

4.5 Roles of Inflammation and Polyamines in Other Cancers

Besides prostate and colon cancer, polyamine metabolism (by use of polyamine synthesis inhibitors or polyamine catabolism activators) and inflammation (by use of NSAIDs) have been studied for many cancers, including skin, lung, bladder (Messing et al. 2006; Herr 2007), cervical (Vlastos et al. 2005), esophageal (Fong et al. 2001), gastric (Takahashi et al. 2000), pancreatic, and breast (Xu et al. 2008). These agents have been used independent of each other and have shown varying results due to the lack of a consensus for the dose and the length of the study. There is compelling evidence that both polyamines and inflammation play a crucial role in these cancers. For example, inflammation has been postulated to play a key role in lung carcinogenesis. There is a growing body of evidence to suggest that smoking induced pulmonary inflammation increases lung cancer development in smokers (Brody and Spira 2006; Smith et al. 2006) and in the regular use of aspirin and other nonsteroidal anti-inflammatory drugs is associated with reduced risk of developing lung cancer in animal models and in smokers (Moysich et al. 2002; Smith et al. 2006). It has been shown that induction of spermine oxidase by a pro-inflammatory cytokine like TNFalpha which is generated due to chronic inflammation, can lead to the continuous production of reactive oxygen species (ROS) which in turn can lead to DNA damage thereby leading to mutations (Babbar and Casero 2006). Further, drugs that decrease the concentrations of intracellular polyamines have been shown to have preventive effects in lung cancer cells, as is the case with polyamine analogs, which increase the polyamine catabolism (Huang et al. 2005) or DFMO which inhibits polyamine synthesis.

The nonmelanoma skin cancers (NMSC), basal cell carcinoma (BCC) and squamous cell carcinoma (SCC), are the most common malignancies in whites worldwide. The vast majority of NMSCs are caused by excessive exposure to UV radiation. BCC and SCC prevention has focused mainly on limiting the amount of UV radiation that reaches the skin. Research into the pathogenesis of BCC and SCC has stimulated interest in chemopreventive agents that inhibit the activity of COX-2 and ODC, both of which contribute to UVB-induced skin cancer development. In murine models as well as in humans, UVB enhances the expression of COX-2-dependent prostaglandin production, particularly of PGE2 (Athar et al. 2001; An et al. 2002; Rundhaug and Fischer 2008). COX-2 and PGE2 have important roles in skin carcinogenesis, stimulating the proliferation of preneoplastic cells and promoting inflammation during the promotion stage. They also facilitate the epithelial-to-mesenchymal transition, suppress host antitumor defense mechanisms, inhibit tumor cell apoptosis, and stimulate angiogenesis during the progression stage of skin carcinogenesis. Not expressed in undamaged normal epidermis, COX-2 can be induced in such tissue by acute and chronic exposure to UVB (Rundhaug and Fischer 2008) and is overexpressed in the epithelia of actinic keratoses and SCCs (An et al. 2002). COX-2 is also found in BCC, where its distribution differs from that of SCCs. COX-2 is found in the stroma surrounding islands of epithelial BCC cells in mice and primarily in the tissue adjacent to BCC islands in humans (An et al. 2002). ODC activity and polyamine levels are dramatically elevated in human squamous cell carcinomas compared to adjacent normal skin tissue. ODC is also transiently induced in the skin by a variety of stimuli including mitogens, tumor promoters such as 12-O-tetradecanoylphorbol ester (TPA), and hormones which has been confirmed by the use of transgenic mouse models for skin tumorigenesis. Several transgenic mouse model studies have shown the essential role of polyamines in the early promotion of skin tumorigenesis. Elevated levels of ODC activity are sufficient to promote skin tumor formation, without the addition of tumor-promoting agents, in the carcinogen-exposed skin of K6/ODC transgenic mice, where ODC is constitutively targeted to the skin with a keratin 6 or keratin 5 promoters (Tang et al. 2004). In addition, doses of UVB radiation that are insufficient to produce tumors in SKH-1 hairless mice will induce both premalignant papillomas and SCCs in K6/ODC transgenic mice. Numerous preclinical studies provide further evidence of the contribution of ODC to the development of BCC is convincing (Tang et al. 2004). DFMO has been shown to have an inhibitory effect on skin carcinogenesis by depleting polyamine levels in murine models of skin cancer (Gensler 1991; Ahmad et al. 2001; Megosh et al. 2002). As recently reported by Bailey et al. a randomized, double-blind, placebo-controlled phase III trial of DFMO (0.5 g/m^2/day) versus placebo for up to 5 years produced promising results in men and women with a previous history of skin cancer (Bailey et al. 2010). Although DFMO did not achieve the primary objective of a statistically significant reduction in new NMSC or inhibit the development of SCC, it decreased BCCs by 30%. The BCC result was significant not only from a statistical standpoint (P=0.03), but also because it is the first time that a chemopreventive agent other than sunscreens has prevented BCCs in subjects who do not have conditions that predispose them to develop this cancer. This study provided evidence that ODC inhibition represents an important molecular target-based approach for preventing skin cancer and validates the utility of DFMO as a cancer chemopreventive agent in another human organ system besides the colon. Fischer et al. showed that treatment with a combination of DFMO and the NSAID celecoxib was more effective in diminishing UVB-induced SCCs in murine skin than the treatment with either agent alone (Fischer et al. 2001). These findings coincide nicely with the findings of Meyskens et al. in colorectal adenomatous polyps. Therefore, adding an oral COX inhibitor to oral DFMO may have additive or synergistic effects in BCC and may allow chemopreventive efficacy with a lower dose of DFMO and/or the COX inhibitor, thus potentially reducing the toxicity either single agent might cause.

4.6 Conclusions

Recent clinical trials suggest that targeting polyamine metabolism alone or in combination with anti-inflammatory drugs (NSAIDS) is an effective and relatively safe method of reducing risk factors (e.g., colon adenomas for colon cancer, PSA doubling time for prostate cancer) for specific cancers. Experimental evidence suggests that polyamine metabolism may influence inflammatory processes and that certain NSAIDS act on polyamine metabolism by activating polyamine export mechanisms. The strategy of combining polyamine synthesis inhibitors with NSAIDS may be applicable for reduction of risk factors for several major types of human cancer.

Disclaimer The views and opinions presented by Babbar, N. are solely the author's and do not necessarily reflect the views and opinions of his employer, Osmetech Molecular Diagnostics.

Acknowledgments This work was supported in part by grants from the USPHS National Institutes of Health CA95060 and CA123065.

References

Ahmad N, Gilliam AC, Katiyar SK et al (2001) A definitive role of ornithine decarboxylase in photocarcinogenesis. Am J Pathol 159(3):885–892

Alberts DS, Martinez ME, Roe DJ et al (2000) Lack of effect of a high-fiber cereal supplement on the recurrence of colorectal adenomas. Phoenix Colon Cancer Prevention Physicians' Network. N Engl J Med 342(16):1156–1162

An KP, Athar M, Tang X et al (2002) Cyclooxygenase-2 expression in murine and human nonmelanoma skin cancers: implications for therapeutic approaches. Photochem Photobiol 76(1):73–80

Arber N, Eagle CJ, Spicak J et al (2006) Celecoxib for the prevention of colorectal adenomatous polyps. N Engl J Med 355(9):885–895

Athar M, An KP, Morel KD et al (2001) Ultraviolet B(UVB)-induced cox-2 expression in murine skin: an immunohistochemical study. Biochem Biophys Res Commun 280(4):1042–1047

Babbar N, Casero RA Jr (2006) Tumor necrosis factor-alpha increases reactive oxygen species by inducing spermine oxidase in human lung epithelial cells: a potential mechanism for inflammation-induced carcinogenesis. Cancer Res 66(23):11125–11130

Babbar N, Ignatenko NA, Casero RA Jr et al (2003) Cyclooxygenase-independent induction of apoptosis by sulindac sulfone is mediated by polyamines in colon cancer. J Biol Chem 278(48): 47762–47775

Babbar N, Gerner EW, Casero RA Jr (2006) Induction of spermidine/spermine N1-acetyltransferase (SSAT) by aspirin in Caco-2 colon cancer cells. Biochem J 394(Pt 1):317–324

Babbar N, Murray-Stewart T, Casero RA Jr (2007) Inflammation and polyamine catabolism: the good, the bad and the ugly. Biochem Soc Trans 35(Pt 2):300–304

Bailey HH, Kim K, Verma AK et al (2010) A randomized, double-blind, placebo-controlled phase 3 skin cancer prevention study of {alpha}-difluoromethylornithine in subjects with previous history of skin cancer. Cancer Prev Res (Phila Pa) 3(1):35–47

Balkwill F, Mantovani A (2001) Inflammation and cancer: back to Virchow? Lancet 357(9255):539–545

Bardia A, Platz EA, Yegnasubramanian S et al (2009) Anti-inflammatory drugs, antioxidants, and prostate cancer prevention. Curr Opin Pharmacol 9(4):419–426

Baron JA, Beach M, Mandel JS et al (1999) Calcium supplements for the prevention of colorectal adenomas. Calcium Polyp Prevention Study Group. N Engl J Med 340(2):101–107

Baron JA, Cole BF, Sandler RS et al (2003) A randomized trial of aspirin to prevent colorectal adenomas. N Engl J Med 348(10):891–899

Baron JA, Sandler RS, Bresalier RS et al (2006) A randomized trial of rofecoxib for the chemoprevention of colorectal adenomas. Gastroenterology 131(6):1674–1682

Barry EL, Baron JA, Bhat S et al (2006) Ornithine decarboxylase polymorphism modification of response to aspirin treatment for colorectal adenoma prevention. J Natl Cancer Inst 98(20):1494–1500

Bernstein H, Holubec H, Bernstein C et al (2006) Unique dietary-related mouse model of colitis. Inflamm Bowel Dis 12(4):278–293

Bernstein H, Holubec H, Bernstein C et al (2007) Deoxycholate-induced colitis is markedly attenuated in Nos2 knockout mice in association with modulation of gene expression profiles. Dig Dis Sci 52(3):628–642

Bertagnolli MM, Eagle CJ, Zauber AG et al (2006) Celecoxib for the prevention of sporadic colorectal adenomas. N Engl J Med 355(9):873–884

Bettuzzi S, Davalli P, Astancolle S et al (2000) Tumor progression is accompanied by significant changes in the levels of expression of polyamine metabolism regulatory genes and clusterin (sulfated glycoprotein 2) in human prostate cancer specimens. Cancer Res 60(1):28–34

Block TM, Mehta AS, Fimmel CJ et al (2003) Molecular viral oncology of hepatocellular carcinoma. Oncogene 22(33):5093–5107

Brody JS, Spira A (2006) State of the art. Chronic obstructive pulmonary disease, inflammation, and lung cancer. Proc Am Thorac Soc 3(6):535–537

Coleman CS, Stanley BA, Viswanath R et al (1994) Rapid exchange of subunits of mammalian ornithine decarboxylase. J Biol Chem 269(5): 3155–3158

Coussens LM, Werb Z (2002) Inflammation and cancer. Nature 420(6917):860–867

Crozat A, Palvimo JJ, Julkunen M et al (1992) Comparison of androgen regulation of ornithine decarboxylase and S-adenosylmethionine decarboxylase gene expression in rodent kidney and accessory sex organs. Endocrinology 130(3): 1131–1144

Cyriac J, Haleem R, Cai X et al (2002) Androgen regulation of spermidine synthase expression in the rat prostate. Prostate 50(4):252–261

Danzin C, Jung MJ, Claverie N et al (1979) Effects of alpha-difluoromethylornithine, an enzyme-activated irreversible inhibitor or ornithine decarboxylase, on testosterone-induced regeneration of prostate and seminal vesicle in castrated rats. Biochem J 180(3):507–513

4

De Marzo AM, Nakai Y, Nelson WG (2007a) Inflammation, atrophy, and prostate carcinogenesis. Urol Oncol 25(5):398–400

De Marzo AM, Platz EA, Sutcliffe S et al (2007b) Inflammation in prostate carcinogenesis. Nat Rev Cancer 7(4):256–269

Deutsch ME (1992) Aspirin use and reduced risk of fatal colon cancer. N Engl J Med 326(19):1289; discussion 1290–1281

Elitsur Y, Moshier JA, Murthy R et al (1992) Polyamine levels, ornithine decarboxylase (ODC) activity, and ODC-mRNA expression in normal and cancerous human colonocytes. Life Sci 50(19):1417–1424

Erdman SH, Ignatenko NA, Powell MB et al (1999) APC-dependent changes in expression of genes influencing polyamine metabolism, and consequences for gastrointestinal carcinogenesis, in the Min mouse. Carcinogenesis 20(9):1709–1713

Fearon ER, Vogelstein B (1990) A genetic model for colorectal tumorigenesis. Cell 61(5):759–767

Fischer SM, Lee M, Lubet RA (2001) Difluoromethylornithine is effective as both a preventive and therapeutic agent against the development of UV carcinogenesis in SKH hairless mice. Carcinogenesis 22(1):83–88

Fjosne HE, Strand H, Sunde A (1992) Dose-dependent induction of ornithine decarboxylase and S-adenosyl-methionine decarboxylase activity by testosterone in the accessory sex organs of male rats. Prostate 21(3):239–245

Fong LY, Nguyen VT, Pegg AE et al (2001) Alpha-difluoromethylornithine induction of apoptosis: a mechanism which reverses pre-established cell proliferation and cancer initiation in esophageal carcinogenesis in zinc-deficient rats. Cancer Epidemiol Biomarkers Prev 10(3):191–199

Fultz KE, Gerner EW (2002) APC-dependent regulation of ornithine decarboxylase in human colon tumor cells. Mol Carcinog 34(1):10–18

Gensler HL (1991) Prevention by alpha-difluoromethylornithine of skin carcinogenesis and immunosuppression induced by ultraviolet irradiation. J Cancer Res Clin Oncol 117(4):345–350

Gerner EW, Garewal HS, Emerson SS et al (1994) Gastrointestinal tissue polyamine contents of patients with Barrett's esophagus treated with alpha-difluoromethylornithine. Cancer Epidemiol Biomarkers Prev 3(4):325–330

Gerner EW, Ignatenko NA, Besselsen DG (2003). Preclinical models for chemoprevention of colon cancer. Recent Results Cancer Res 163:58–71; discussion 264–266

Giardiello FM, Hamilton SR, Krush AJ et al (1993) Treatment of colonic and rectal adenomas with sulindac in familial adenomatous polyposis. N Engl J Med 328(18):1313–1316

Giardiello FM, Hamilton SR, Hylind LM et al (1997) Ornithine decarboxylase and polyamines in familial adenomatous polyposis. Cancer Res 57(2):199–201

Gobert AP, Cheng Y, Wang JY et al (2002) Helicobacter pylori induces macrophage apoptosis by activation of arginase II. J Immunol 168(9):4692–4700

Goldberg Y (1996) Aspirin and colon cancer. N Engl J Med 334(12):800–801

Goodwin AC, Jadallah S, Toubaji A et al (2008) Increased spermine oxidase expression in human prostate cancer and prostatic intraepithelial neoplasia tissues. Prostate 68(7):766–772

Greenberg ER, Baron JA, Freeman DH Jr et al (1993) Reduced risk of large-bowel adenomas among aspirin users. The Polyp Prevention Study Group. J Natl Cancer Inst 85(11):912–916

Gupta S, Ahmad N, Marengo SR et al (2000) Chemoprevention of prostate carcinogenesis by alpha-difluoromethylornithine in TRAMP mice. Cancer Res 60(18):5125–5133

Halline AG, Brasitus TA (1990) Effect of PAO inhibition on the colonic malignant transformation process induced by 1, 2-dimethylhydrazine. Carcinogenesis 11:2127–2132

Hanahan D, Weinberg RA (2000) The hallmarks of cancer. Cell 100(1):57–70

Hayashi S, Murakami Y, Matsufuji S (1996) Ornithine decarboxylase antizyme: a novel type of regulatory protein. Trends Biochem Sci 21(1):27–30

Herr HW (2007) Does difluoromethylornithine prevent recurrence in low-risk superficial bladder cancer? Nat Clin Pract Urol 4(5):240–241

Higuchi CM, Wang W (1995) Comodulation of cellular polyamines and proliferation: biomarker application to colorectal mucosa. J Cell Biochem 57(2):256–261

Hixson LJ, Garewal HS, McGee DL et al (1993) Ornithine decarboxylase and polyamines in colorectal neoplasia and mucosa. Cancer Epidemiol Biomarkers Prev 2(4):369–374

Huang Y, Pledgie A, Casero RA Jr et al (2005) Molecular mechanisms of polyamine analogs in cancer cells. Anticancer Drugs 16(3): 229–241

Hubner RA, Muir KR, Liu JF et al (2008) Ornithine decarboxylase G316A genotype is prognostic for colorectal adenoma recurrence and predicts

efficacy of aspirin chemoprevention. Clin Cancer Res 14(8):2303–2309
Ignatenko NA, Babbar N, Mehta D et al (2004) Suppression of polyamine catabolism by activated Ki-ras in human colon cancer cells. Mol Carcinog 39(2):91–102
Ignatenko NA, Besselsen DG, Roy UK et al (2006) Dietary putrescine reduces the intestinal anticarcinogenic activity of sulindac in a murine model of familial adenomatous polyposis. Nutr Cancer 56(2):172–181
Jacobs EJ, Rodriguez C, Mondul AM et al (2005) A large cohort study of aspirin and other nonsteroidal anti-inflammatory drugs and prostate cancer incidence. J Natl Cancer Inst 97(13):975–980
Kee K, Foster BA, Merali S et al (2004) Activated polyamine catabolism depletes acetyl-CoA pools and suppresses prostate tumor growth in TRAMP mice. J Biol Chem 279(38):40076–40083
Lawson KR, Ignatenko NA, Piazza GA et al (2000) Influence of K-ras activation on the survival responses of Caco-2 cells to the chemopreventive agents sulindac and difluoromethylornithine. Cancer Epidemiol Biomarkers Prev 9(11):1155–1162
Li H, Schut HA, Conran P et al (1999) Prevention by aspirin and its combination with alpha-difluoromethylornithine of azoxymethane-induced tumors, aberrant crypt foci and prostaglandin E2 levels in rat colon. Carcinogenesis 20(3):425–430
Loser C, Folsch UR, Paprotny C et al (1990) Polyamines in colorectal cancer. Evaluation of polyamine concentrations in the colon tissue, serum, and urine of 50 patients with colorectal cancer. Cancer 65(4):958–966
Luk GD, Baylin SB (1984) Ornithine decarboxylase as a biologic marker in familial colonic polyposis. N Engl J Med 311(2):80–83
Macarthur M, Hold GL, El-Omar EM (2004) Inflammation and Cancer II. Role of chronic inflammation and cytokine gene polymorphisms in the pathogenesis of gastrointestinal malignancy. Am J Physiol Gastrointest Liver Physiol 286(4):G515–520
Mahmud SM, Tanguay S, Begin LR et al (2006) Non-steroidal anti-inflammatory drug use and prostate cancer in a high-risk population. Eur J Cancer Prev 15(2):158–164
Martinez ME, O'Brien TG, Fultz KE et al (2003) Pronounced reduction in adenoma recurrence associated with aspirin use and a polymorphism in the ornithine decarboxylase gene. Proc Natl Acad Sci U S A 100(13):7859–7864
Megosh LC, Hu J, George K et al (2002) Genetic control of polyamine-dependent susceptibility to skin tumorigenesis. Genomics 79(4):505–512
Messing E, Kim KM, Sharkey F et al (2006) Randomized prospective phase III trial of difluoromethylornithine vs placebo in preventing recurrence of completely resected low risk superficial bladder cancer. J Urol 176(2): 500–504
Meyskens FL Jr, McLaren CE, Pelot D et al (2008) Difluoromethylornithine plus sulindac for the prevention of sporadic colorectal adenomas: a randomized placebo-controlled, double-blind trial. Cancer Prev Res (Phila Pa) 1(1):32–38
Mohan RR, Challa A, Gupta S et al (1999) Overexpression of ornithine decarboxylase in prostate cancer and prostatic fluid in humans. Clin Cancer Res 5(1):143–147
Moysich KB, Menezes RJ, Ronsani A et al (2002) Regular aspirin use and lung cancer risk. BMC Cancer 2:31
Nigro ND, Bull AW, Boyd ME (1986) Inhibition of intestinal carcinogenesis in rats: effect of difluoromethylornithine with piroxicam or fish oil. J Natl Cancer Inst 77(6):1309–1313
Paganini-Hill A, Hsu G, Ross RK et al (1992). Aspirin use and reduced risk of fatal colon cancer. N Engl J Med 326(19):1290; discussion 1290–1291.
Parker MT, Gerner EW (2002) Polyamine-mediated post-transcriptional regulation of COX-2. Biochimie 84(8):815–819
Risch HA, Howe GR (1995) Pelvic inflammatory disease and the risk of epithelial ovarian cancer. Cancer Epidemiol Biomarkers Prev 4(5):447–451
Rundhaug JE, Fischer SM (2008) Cyclooxygenase-2 plays a critical role in UV-induced skin carcinogenesis. Photochem Photobiol 84(2): 322–329
Russell D, Snyder SH (1968) Amine synthesis in rapidly growing tissues: ornithine decarboxylase activity in regenerating rat liver, chick embryo, and various tumors. Proc Natl Acad Sci U S A 60(4):1420–1427
Sandler RS, Halabi S, Baron JA et al (2003) A randomized trial of aspirin to prevent colorectal adenomas in patients with previous colorectal cancer. N Engl J Med 348(10):883–890
Schatzkin A, Lanza E, Corle D et al (2000) Lack of effect of a low-fat, high-fiber diet on the recurrence of colorectal adenomas. Polyp Prevention Trial Study Group. N Engl J Med 342(16):1149–1155

4

Schipper RG, Deli G, Deloyer P et al (2000) Antitumor activity of the polyamine analog N(1), N(11)-diethylnorspermine against human prostate carcinoma cells. Prostate 44(4):313–321

Schreinemachers DM, Everson RB (1994) Aspirin use and lung, colon, and breast cancer incidence in a prospective study. Epidemiology 5(2):138–146

Seiler N (1987) Functions of polyamine acetylation. Can J Physiol Pharmacol 65(10):2024–2035

Simoneau AR, Gerner EW, Nagle R et al (2008) The effect of difluoromethylornithine on decreasing prostate size and polyamines in men: results of a year-long phase IIb randomized placebo-controlled chemoprevention trial. Cancer Epidemiol Biomarkers Prev 17(2):292–299

Smith CJ, Perfetti TA, King JA (2006) Perspectives on pulmonary inflammation and lung cancer risk in cigarette smokers. Inhal Toxicol 18(9):667–677

Solomon SD, Pfeffer MA, McMurray JJ et al (2006) Effect of celecoxib on cardiovascular events and blood pressure in two trials for the prevention of colorectal adenomas. Circulation 114(10):1028–1035

Steinbach G, Lynch PM, Phillips RK et al (2000) The effect of celecoxib, a cyclooxygenase-2 inhibitor, in familial adenomatous polyposis. N Engl J Med 342(26):1946–1952

Stoner GD, Budd GT, Ganapathi R et al (1999) Sulindac sulfone induced regression of rectal polyps in patients with familial adenomatous polyposis. Adv Exp Med Biol 470:45–53

Takahashi Y, Mai M, Nishioka K (2000) alpha-difluoromethylornithine induces apoptosis as well as anti-angiogenesis in the inhibition of tumor growth and metastasis in a human gastric cancer model. Int J Cancer 85(2):243–247

Tang X, Kim AL, Feith DJ et al (2004) Ornithine decarboxylase is a target for chemoprevention of basal and squamous cell carcinomas in Ptch1+/- mice. J Clin Invest 113(6):867–875

ter Steege JC, Forget PP, Buurman WA (1999) Oral spermine administration inhibits nitric oxide-mediated intestinal damage and levels of systemic inflammatory mediators in a mouse endotoxin model. Shock 11(2):115–119

Thomas T, Thomas TJ (2001) Polyamines in cell growth and cell death: molecular mechanisms and therapeutic applications. Cell Mol Life Sci 58(2):244–258

Thun MJ, Namboodiri MM, Heath CW Jr (1991) Aspirin use and reduced risk of fatal colon cancer. N Engl J Med 325(23):1593–1596

Uemura T, Yerushalmi HF, Tsaprailis G et al (2008) Identification and characterization of a diamine exporter in colon epithelial cells. J Biol Chem 283(39):26428–26435

Vesterinen E, Pukkala E, Timonen T et al (1993) Cancer incidence among 78,000 asthmatic patients. Int J Epidemiol 22(6):976–982

Visvanathan K, Helzlsouer KJ, Boorman DW et al (2004) Association among an ornithine decarboxylase polymorphism, androgen receptor gene (CAG) repeat length and prostate cancer risk. J Urol 171(2 Pt 1):652–655

Vlastos AT, West LA, Atkinson EN et al (2005) Results of a phase II double-blinded randomized clinical trial of difluoromethylornithine for cervical intraepithelial neoplasia grades 2 to 3. Clin Cancer Res 11(1):390–396

Wang JY, Johnson LR, Tsai YH et al (1991) Mucosal ornithine decarboxylase, polyamines, and hyperplasia in infected intestine. Am J Physiol 260(1 Pt 1):G45–51

Whitcomb DC (2004) Inflammation and Cancer V. Chronic pancreatitis and pancreatic cancer. Am J Physiol Gastrointest Liver Physiol 287(2):G315–319

Xu H, Chaturvedi R, Cheng Y et al (2004) Spermine oxidation induced by Helicobacter pylori results in apoptosis and DNA damage: implications for gastric carcinogenesis. Cancer Res 64(23): 8521–8525

Xu H, Washington S, Verderame MF et al (2008) Role of non-receptor and receptor tyrosine kinases (TKs) in the antitumor action of alpha-difluoromethylornithine (DFMO) in breast cancer cells. Breast Cancer Res Treat 112(2): 255–261

Yerushalmi HF, Besselsen DG, Ignatenko NA et al (2006a) The role of NO synthases in arginine-dependent small intestinal and colonic carcinogenesis. Mol Carcinog 45(2):93–105

Yerushalmi HF, Besselsen DG, Ignatenko NA et al (2006b) Role of polyamines in arginine-dependent colon carcinogenesis in Apc(Min) (/+) mice. Mol Carcinog 45(10):764–773

Zell AJ, Pelot D, Chen WP et al. (2009). "Risk of cardiovascular events in a randomized placebo-controlled, double blind trial of difluoromethylornithine plus sulindac for the prevention of sporadic colorectal adenomas." Cancer Prev Res (Phila Pa) 2(3): 209–212.

Zhang M, Caragine T, Wang H et al (1997) Spermine inhibits proinflammatory cytokine synthesis in human mononuclear cells: a counterregulatory mechanism that restrains the immune response. J Exp Med 185(10):1759–1768

Thinking About the Role (Largely Ignored) of Heavy Metals in Cancer Prevention: Hexavalent Chromium and Melanoma as a Case in Point

5

Frank L. Meyskens and Sun Yang

Abstract Ultraviolet (UV) light exposure accounts for only 40–50% of the attributable risk for cutaneous melanoma (CM); also classical UV-induced lesions are rare in melanomas (especially among CM with NRAS or BRAF mutations). It is therefore likely that an additional environmental factor exists as familial and genetic factors play a role in less than 5%. A large amount of (largely forgotten) epidemiologic data indicates that heavy metal exposure is strongly associated with the development of CM. Also, epidemiologic studies of patients with joint replacement indicate a marked subsequent time-related increase in melanoma in patients with metal-on-metal hip arthroplasties. In these patients chromium and cobalt levels rise to10x normal and stay elevated at levels two- to threefold normal for at least 10 years. Chromium is widely used in industry for its anticorrosive and steel-strengthening properties and is widespread in everyday materials. Our hypothesis is therefore that chromium, alone or in conjunction with UV, plays a major role in the pathogenesis of CM. We have incubated human neonatal melanocytes for more than 10 weeks in the presence of a wide range and concentrations of metals without effect except by hexavalent chromium Cr(VI)and to a lesser degree Co^{2+}. After prolonged culture, chromium-incubated cells produced foci and when replated secondary colonies formed. We have just begun to study this phenomenon in more detail and studies without and with different wavelengths of UV will be explored. Of interest is that aneuploidy (a universal chromosomal change in cutaneous melanoma) in lymphocytes in patients with hip-on-hip metal prostheses has been demonstrated by others.

F.L. Meyskens (✉) and S. Yang
Departments of Medicine,
University of California, Irvine
Biological Chemistry, University of California, Irvine, and
Chao Family Comprehensive Cancer Center,
University of California, Irvine, CA, USA
e-mail: flmeyske@uci.edu

5.1 Background

5.1.1 The Evolution of the Idea

University of California, Irvine was one of the clinical sites for the conduct of the β-carotene and retinol trial (CARET) to prevent lung cancer in smokers. The results were shocking: patients supplemented with high doses of β-carotene

H.-J. Senn and F. Otto (eds.), *Clinical Cancer Prevention*,
Recent Results in Cancer Research 188, DOI: 10.1007/978-3-642-10858-7_5,

5

developed more rather than fewer lung cancers (Omenn et al. 1996). The overall conclusion had to be: an antioxidant could act as a pro-oxidant in the clinical setting. This observation led me to take a sabbatical with a world-class oxidant chemist (Helmut Sies, Düsseldorf, Germany). Subsequently, my basic laboratory work on CM has been driven by two vexing clinical observations:

1. *Why is nonmelanoma skin cancer common and melanoma rare in black or white albinos?* After nearly 10 years worth of work, mainly with organic chemist Pat Farmer, these studies led to the recognition that melanomagenesis is a redox-driven process (Meyskens et al. 2001a, b; Gidanian et al. 2008) and that this process could be co-opted to develop new therapies for melanoma, observations translated by us and others (Fruehauf and Meyskens 2007).
2. *Why are melanomas more common in patients with metal-on-metal hip replacements?* Although this finding was initially made over 15 years ago (Nyren et al. 1995), recognition of its potential broader importance was missed by us and others until a large meta-analysis (Onega et al. 2006) demonstrated that melanoma was increased in patients with metal-on-metal hip replacements. This observation plus our growing interest in redox-changes in melanin during melanomagenesis inevitably led to the question: *could metals contribute to the pathogenesis of cutaneous melanoma?*

5.1.2 Substances That Bind Melanin

5.1.2.1 Metals

It has been known for some time that metals bind melanin (Sarna et al. 1976; Crippa et al. 1989; Hong et al. 2004; Hong and Simon 2007), the major differentiation product of melanocytes. A summary of metals known to bind melanin is provided in Table 5.1. Although the biochemistry and chemistry of melanin, with two major forms, eumelanin and pleomelanin, is very complex (Simon et al. 2009) the simple concept is that when reduced melanin (usual state) is partially oxidized, the metal bound to melanin serves as a low-grade superoxide generator with downstream effects on signaling pathways (Meyskens et al. 2001a, b). We have discussed elsewhere the importance of free Cu^{2+} and Fe^{2+} contributing, respectively, to oxidative stress during melanosomal disruption that accompanies the process of melanomagenesis (Gidanian et al. 2008) and during sub-burn-induced angiogenesis and the release of free hemoglobin-Fe (Meyskens and Berwick 2008). Of related interest is that we have known for some time that the imaging compound $^{67}Ga^{III}$ (an Fe ^{III} analog) binds avidly to the melanin in melanoma patients. However, we will not delve further into the issue of the importance of free iron and copper during melanomagenesis as Cr(VI) is the focus of this essay.

Table 5.1 Possible metals as pro-carcinogens in melanomogenesis

Metals that have been identified in natural melanins
Biometals Cu, Zn, Fe
Trace biometals Ni, Mo, Mn, Co
Nonbiological Cr, Au, Ag, Pb
Promotion of OH predicted for
• *Redox active metals*
Cu, Fe, Cr,Mn, Co,Pb
• *Increase in semiquinone radical*
Sc3+, La3+, In3+, Al3+, Zn2+, Cd2+

5.1.2.2 Nonmetals

A wide variety of other nonmetal substances bind melanin including most notably a variety of insecticides and polychlorinated biphenyls (generated in electrical situations). Other nonmetal-binding substances include thioureas (food preservatives) and various other organic compounds including β-blockers, alpha-agonists, antibiotics, antimaterials, organic amines, and polycyclic aromatic hydrocarbons. Interestingly, melanin was also found to be bound with different chemotherapeutic agents such as Doxorubicin (900 nmol/mg) and daunorubicin (760 nmol/mg), which was associated with the development of drug resistance (Svensson et al. 2003; Chen et al. 2006).

5.2 Major Risk Factors for Cutaneous Melanoma

5.2.1 Epidemiology

5.2.1.1 Sunlight

Numerous studies from several countries have implicated exposure to sunlight (ultraviolet light radiation or UV) as a causative agent in the development of nonmelanoma (NMSC) and CM skin cancer (Berwick and Wiggins 2006; Maddodi and Setaluri 2008; review Abdel-Malek et al. 2010). However, the details are quite different. NMSC is associated with cumulative lifetime UV exposure. In contrast, melanoma is associated with prepubertal and intermittent adult sunburns, especially in individuals who have type I and type II skin and hence burn easily. *How could that work? How biologically would a sunburn at age 12 translate to a melanoma 20, 30, 40 years later?*

Another unique feature is that NMSC consistently exhibits evidence of UV damage, i.e., classical pyrimidine dimers. In contrast such damage is rarely detected in primary horizontal growth phase melanomas although a distinct set of genetic alterations are found (Curtin et al. 2005) in which genomic instability is already evident (Hussein et al. 2005). During vertical growth phase, and subsequently, metastatic disease shows extensive aneuploidy, a chromosomal abnormality somewhat unique to CM. Of related interest is the recent complete genomic sequencing of a metastatic melanoma and the cataloging of mutations with an imprint of past UV-induced DNA damage *and* evidence of independent mechanisms of damage, including most notably selective application of DNA repair to transcribed genomic regions and evidence of G→T changes as being common (Pleasance et al. 2010). These genomic results strongly suggest that UV is only one player in the pathogenesis of CM and that other cocarcinogens are at work either in conjunction with UV-induced damage or as a parallel operator in producing DNA damage.

5.2.1.2 Occupational Epidemiology

The first review of this topic appeared over 20 years ago (Austin and Reynolds 1986) and suggested a general role for metals in melanoma pathogenesis. Many studies have appeared since. Major studies that demonstrate an increased risk of melanoma for printers/lithographers, electrical workers, and insecticides are briefly summarized in Table 5.2. What is remarkable about these occupational epidemiology studies is that only an increase in CM was found and that no increase for any other cancer was detected.

5.2.1.3 Melanoma After Total Joint Arthroplasty

The field of joint replacement has been concerned for quite some time about the effect of shed metals from arthroplastic devices, with

5

Table 5.2 Occupational epidemiology of cutaneous melanoma

Reference	Cohort	Risk for melanoma
Printers/Lithographers (metals)		
Dubrow 1986	(1968–78) 577	PMR460(p=0.01)
(RI)[a] Nielson 1996	(b 1933–42) 837	RR 3.4
(Danish) Bouchardy 2002	(d 1968–78) 262	OR 1.6
(Swiss) Perez 2004	(1971–89) 1.8M (6,187 melanoma)	RR 2.8
Electrical Workers (polychlorinated biphenyls)		
Loomis 1997	Retrospective 138, 905	RR 1.23–1.71 dose response 1.29–4.8 (10 year)
Sinks 1992	Retrospective 3,588	8 years 2 expected (SMR 4.1)
Clapp 206 (US)	31,941 decedents	PCMR 179 (131–244)
Nichols 1999 (GB)	>1,000 workers	SMR 221
Ruder 2006	3,569 workers	SMR2.43 (1.1–4.6)
Pest control (insecticides)		
Macfarlane 2009	Pest control workers, Mortality and CA (1980–2000)	SIR 1.56 (1.03–2.37)
Mahajan 2007	Commercial pesticide Carbamate 21,126 workers, 1,291 cases	RR 4.11 (1.33–12.75)UV adjusted
Fortes 2007	Residential pesticide 287 cases, 299 controls	OR 2.18 (1.07–4.43)UV adjusted dose response

[a]RI, Rhode Island

the major initial concern being local sarcomas (review, Learmonth and Case 2007; IARC 1999; Keegan et al. 2008). However, two large studies (Nyren et al. 1995; Visuri et al. 2006) and a very extensive meta-analysis (Onega et al. 2006) have demonstrated an unexpected result. CM was increased post metal-on-metal hip replacements, an increase that parallels levels of chromium in the bloodstream and urine (Heisel et al. 2005). Confirming the importance of these observations was no increase in hip metal-on-plastic or knee (no direct metal contact) arthroplasties. Not unexpectedly, since Cr(VI) is excreted via the kidney, there was an increase in renal cancer, but no evidence of dose–response effect (which is consistent with many studies of chromium pharmokinetics and urinary damage (Onega et al. 2006)). Several studies have shown that Cr(VI) and cobalt increases to ten and fivefold normal, respectively in the first 2 years after implantation and remain elevated (two- to threefold) for over 10 years (Skipor et al. 2002; Dunstan et al. 2005; Ladon et al. 2004).

A logical question then: *Is there evidence of DNA damage from this release of these insoluble and soluble materials (ions and particles) into the blood stream?*

Papageorgious et al. (2007) has demonstrated the genotoxic effects of particles of the alloy on human cells in vitro. No one has looked at the skin (see below) yet, but Ladon et al. (2004) have demonstrated chromosomal aberrations in peripheral blood leukocytes after metal-on-metal hip arthroplasty.

5.3 Metals

5.3.1 Chemistry and Genetic Damage

The biochemistry and chemistry of metal-induced oxidative stress, downstream effects, and carcinogenesis are extremely complex (Leonard et al. 2004; O'Brien et al. 2003; Beyersmann and Hartwig 2008). Although both Cu^{2+} and Fe^{2+}/Fe^{3+} probably play a role in the ongoing pathogenesis of melanoma, the emphasis in this chapter is on the externally introduced metal hexavalent chromium, which as an anticorrosive and a steel strengthener is literally everywhere including the groundwater. The Department of Defense has actually been concerned about this issue for quite some time (Young 2009). Some of the sources of Cr(VI) and materials which contain it are shown in Table 5.3.

Chromium-6 is currently regulated under the 50-micrograms per liter (μg/L) maximum contaminant level (MCL) for total chromium, which equals to 0.05 parts per million (ppm) (http://www.cdph.ca.gov/CERTLIC/DRINKINGWATER/Pages/Chromium6.aspx). In August 2009, the Office of Environmental Health Hazard Assessment (OEHHA) of the California Environmental Protection Agency announced a draft technical support document for hexavalent chromium in drinking water, indicating a new risk assessment and stressing arising concerns of ingested Cr(VI). A PHG of 0.06 ug/L or 0.06 parts per billion (ppb) is proposed for hexavalent chromium in drinking water, based on tumor incidence data from rodent cancer bioassays.

Table 5.3 Sources and human exposure of chromium Cr(VI), an anticorrosive and a steel strengthener

Chromate manufacture	Joint replacements
Catalytic convertors	Orthodontics
Chrome plating	Razor blades
Stainless steel welding	Blownupsteelstructures–e.g., 9–11, Iraq

5.3.2 Chromium Chemistry

The chemistry of chromium is certainly the most complex of all metals and affects cells in a manner, for the most part, *not* driven by the production of oxo-8-dG lesions, but by a diversity of other effects including interruption of topoisomerase DNA binding which leads to infidelity in replication (Snow 1991).

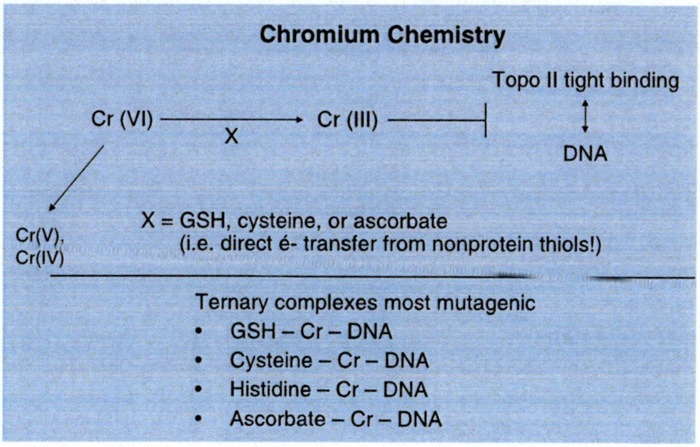

A unique feature of chromium chemistry is that during the reduction of Cr(V1) to Cr(III), highly mutagenic ternary complexes are formed within cells, and in the attempt to repair this damage, aneuploidy results. Most recently, Arakawa et al. (2006 demonstrated that Cr(III)-DNA adducts induce mainly G → T mutations, which is evident in Pleasance's report with melanoma genomic study.

Chromium Chemistry & Aneuroploidy

*MMR Lost ⟶ *MSI ⟶ *DSB ⟶ aneuroploidy

Cr – DNA damage removed by NER but MMR outcompetes beneficial repair and produces chromosomal breaks

*MMR, mismatch repair; MSI, microsatellite instability, DB, double strand breaks

The remarkable aspect of this process is that 8-oxo-dG damage does not occur, p53 is not inactivated, and G/C pairs are the major target. The overall consequence is that aneuploidy and an ever-evolving mutator phenotype result. We propose that the carcinogenesis of melanocyte transformation may follow the path below (also see Meyskens and Berwick 2008).

(a) *Sunlight*: (UV) → classical pyrimidine dimmers → 8-oxo-dG lesions
(b) *Sunburn* (angiogenesis): free Fe^{2+}/$Fe+^{3}$ recycling, OH•, OH^{-} → more 8-oxo-dG lesions
(c) *External exposure* (melanin binding): Cr(VI) → Cr(III) aneuroploidy
(d) *Progression, melanosomal damage*: free Co^{2+} → OH•, OH^{-}

The first comprehensive study detailing the mutational spectrum of chromium (VI) in human cells was done by Chen and Thilly (1994) on the exon 3 of hypoxanthine guanine phosphoribosyl transferase (hprt) gene. They found four Cr(VI)-induced hotspots within the target sequence: C:G → A:T (4.5% of mutants); A:T → T:A (2.0%); G:C → A:T(2.5%); and C:G → T:A(4.0%). Notably, these differed markedly from that observed with H_2O_2, molecular oxygen, iron (II), or Copper (I)/(II), which are all thought to be dependent on and proceeded via oxygen-free radicals intermediates.

5.3.3 Upregulation of Metallothioneins (MTs)

A key question is: *how do metals get into cells.* In the past decade it has been apparent that a whole family of metal-handling proteins exist to protect cells from free metals (Ekschlager et al. 2009). Weinlich et al. (2006) demonstrated that

- MTS were overexpressed in melanoma cells.
- The percent of cells (and amount) with MTs increase with depth of the primary lesion.
- Presence of MTs predicted progression (RR 2.9, $p < 0.02$ and survival (RR4.1, $p < 0.001$).
- Presence of MTs predicted aggressive disease for thin melanomas.

To date no studies have been reported on the levels of MTs or SNPs of MTs and melanoma risk, but such results would be of great interest.

5.3.4 Some Preliminary Experimental Data

5.3.4.1 Effects of Metals on Human Melanocytes

What is the effect of metals on melanocytes? To date we have done several preliminary experiments, the results of one which are shown in Fig. 5.1.

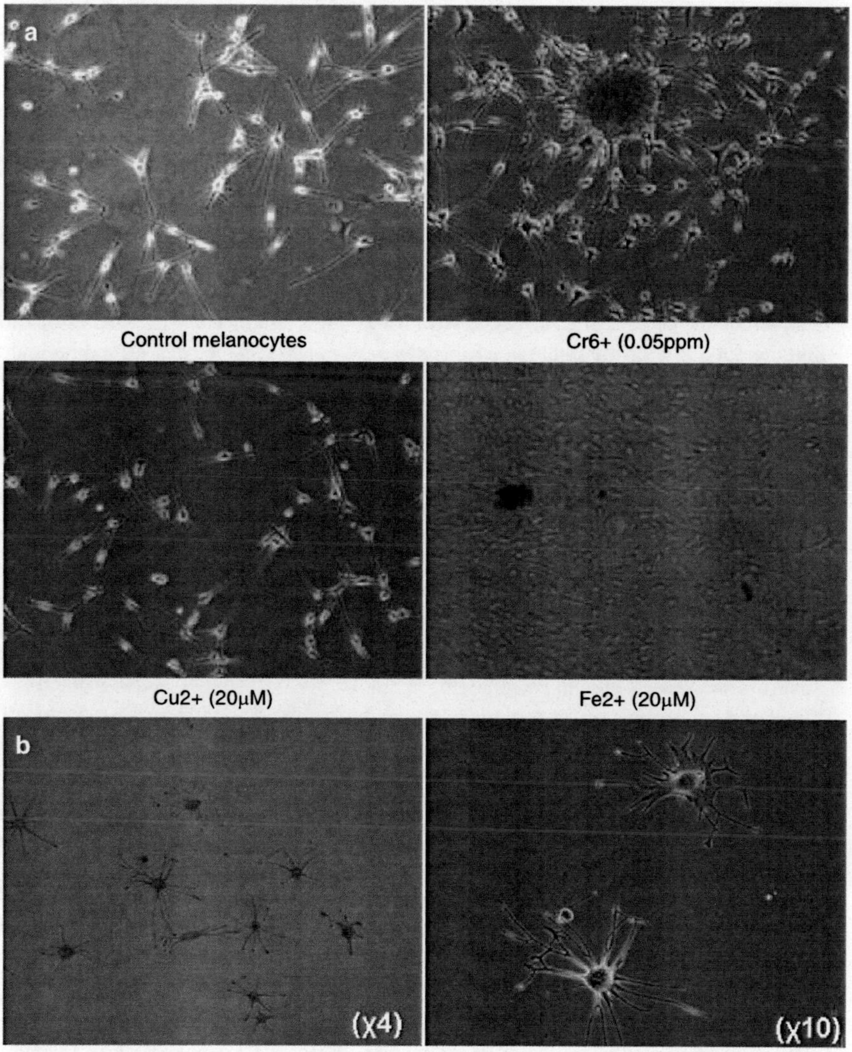

Fig. 5.1 Effects of different metals on human primary melanocytes growth. (**a**): Primary normal melanocytes were cultured in MCDB medium with different metals ($CrCl_6$, $CuCl_2$, and $FeSO_4$) for more than 10 weeks. Cells were passaged once a week and fresh media containing different metals were replaced three times a week. Foci were found in Cr^{6+} (0.05 ppm)-treated cells. After separation and re-passage, cells still form foci in culture dish even at low density. After 10 weeks, photos were taken with control, Cu^{2+} (20 μM) and Fe^{2+} (20 μM) treatments. (**b**): Melanocytes exposed to Cr^{6+} (0.5 ppm) exhibited more dentric-shaped morphologic changes. *Left*, ×40; *Right*, ×100 magnification

Utilizing primary normal melanocytes cultured from human foreskin, we measured the effects of different metals on cell growth including Cr(VI) (0.05 and 0.5 ppm), Cu^{2+} (20 μM), or Fe^{2+} (20 μM) for at least 10 weeks. As shown, all tested metals and dosages exhibited no notable toxicities in melanocytes even after a long-term exposure except Cr(VI) at a concentration of 0.5

5

ppm, which is tenfold of the upper limit standardized for drinking water (0.05 ppm) (California Department of Public Health). Cells exposed to Cr(VI) (0.5 ppm) showed a much slower growth rate compared to control and were associated with significant morphologic changes (Fig. 5.1a) – more dentric-shaped with a flatter cell body. Significant slowdown of cell proliferation was noticed within 4 weeks of treatment and even switching back to regular growth medium could not rescue the cells from toxicity. No significant proliferation rate or morphologic changes were observed with Cu^{2+} or Fe^{2+} treatments.

In distinct contrast from the toxic effects of Cr(VI) at 0.5 ppm, a ten times lower dosage of Cr(VI) (0.05 ppm, drinking water standard), produced a strong stimulating effect on melanocyte growth. Notably, after 3–5 weeks, small foci started to occur in culture dishes (Fig. 5.1b). On collecting these foci and replating them separately, we found that even at a very low cell density, cells still formed foci in vitro exhibiting a gain of extra vertical growth potential (Fig. 5.1b). Further detailed analyses of tumorigenicity and malignant transformation are underway now.

Measurement of Chromium in Primary Melanomas

The use of x-ray synchronization radiation (Bohic et al. 2008) should allow measurement of metals in single cells. Chromium has been detected in metastatic melanoma cells (L. Peterson, personal communications 2009) as has iron, but the hard job of measuring metals in primary melanomas remains to be done.

5.4 Future Prospects

Large cohorts of patients are available who have had hip arthroplasty who are being closely followed, particularly in Scandinavian countries and the United Kingdom. The availability of both tumor registries and arthroplasty registries will provide a source of patients to study. We have already established relationships with investigators there and look forward to detailed studies of chromium in patients who have had arthroplasties and subsequently developed melanomas.

The intriguing results from our preliminary experimental data also suggest that detailed biologic and mechanistic studies of chromium and human melanocytes should be highly informative. Perhaps UV-activated chelators can be developed that will remove this toxic metal (Yiakouvaki et al. 2006).

References

Abdel-Malek ZA, Kadekaro AL, Swope VB et al (2010) Stepping up melanocytes to the challenge of UV exposure. Pig Cell Mel Res 23:171–186

Arakawa H, Wu F, Costa M et al (2006) Sequence specificity of Cr(III)-DNA adduct formation in the p53 gene: NGG sequences are preferential adduct-forming sites. Carcinogenesis 27:639–645

Austin DF, Reynolds (1986) Occupation and malignant melanoma of the skin. Recent Results Cancer Res 102:98–107

Berwick M, Wiggins C (2006) The current epidemiology of cutaneous malignant melanoma. Front Biosci 11:1244–1254

Beyersmann D, Hartwig A (2008) Carcinogenic metal compounds: recent insights into molecular and cellular mechanisms. Arch Tox 82:493–512

Bohic S, Murphy K, Paulus W (2008) Intracellular chemical imaging of the developmental phases of human neuromelanin using synchrotron x-ray microspectroscopy. Anal Chem 80:9557–66

Bouchardy C, Schuler G, Minder C (2002) Cancer risk by occupation and socioeconomic group among men – a study by the Association of Swiss Cancer Registries. Scand J Work Environ Health 28:1–88

Clapp RW (2006) Mortality among US employees of a large computer manufacturing company: 1969–2001. Environ Health 5:30–44

Chen J, Thilly WG (1994) Mutational spectrum of chromium Cr(V1) in human cells. Mut Res 323:21–27

Chen KG, Valencia JC, Lai B et al (2006) Melanosomal sequestration of cytotoxic drugs contributes to the intractability of malignant melanomas. Proc Natl Acad Sci USA 103:9903–9907

Crippa R, Horak V, Prota P (1989) Chemistry of melanins in Alkaloids. Academic, New York

Curtin JA, Fridlyland J, Kageshita T et al (2005) Distinct sets of genetic alterations in melahoma. N Engl J Med 353:2135–47

Dubrow R (1986) Malignant melanoma in the printing industry. Am J Ind Med 10:119–26

Dunstan E, Sanghrajka AP, Tilley S et al (2005) Metal ion levels after metal-on-metal proximal femoral replacements. Jour Bone Joint Surg 5:628–631

Ekschlager T, Adam V, Hrabeta J et al (2009) Metallothioneins and cancer. Curr Protein Pep Sci 10:360–375

Fortes C, Mastroeni S, Melchi F et al (2007) The association between residential pesticide use and cutaneous melanoma. Eur J Cancer 43:1066–1075

Fruehauf JP, Meyskens FL (2007) Reactive oxygen species: a breath of life or death? Clin Cancer Res 13:789–94

Gidanian S, Mentelle M, Meyskens F et al (2008) Melanosomal damage in normal human melanocytes inducted by UVB and metal uptake - a basis for the pro-oxidant state of melanoma. Photochem Photobio 84:556–564

Heisel C, Silva M, Skipor AK (2005) The relationship between activity and ions in patients with metal-on-metal bearing hip Ppostheses. J Bone Joint Sur An 87:781–787

Hong L, Liu Y, Simon JD (2004) Binding of metal ions to melanin and their effects on the aerobic reactivity. Photochem Photobio 80:477–481

Hong L, Simon JD (2007) Current understanding of the binding sites, capacity, affinity, and biological significance of metals in melanin. J Phys Chem B 111:7938–47

Hussein MR, Haemel Ak, Sudilovsky O (2005) Genomic instability in radial growth phase melanoma cell lines after ultraviolet irradiation. Journal of Clinical Pathology 58:389–396

International Agency for Research on Cancer (IARC) (1999) Surgical implants and other foreign bodies. IARC Monograph 74:303–311

Keegan G, Learmonth I, Case P (2008) A systematic comparison of the actual, potential, and theoretical health effects of cobalt and chromium exposures from industry and surgical implants. Critic Rev Toxicol 38:645–674

Ladon D, Doherty A, Newson R et al (2004) Changes in metal levels and chromosome aberrations in the peripheral blood of patients after metal-on-metal hip arthroplasty. J Arthroplast 19:78–83

Learmonth ID, Case CP (2007) Metallic debris from orthopaedic implants. Lancet 369:542–4

Leonard S, Harris G, Shi X (2004) Metal-induced oxidative stress and signal transduction. Free Rad Biol Med 37:1921–1942

Loomis D, Browing SR, Schenck AP (1997) Mortality among electric utility workers exposed to polychlorinated bipheryls. Occup Environ Med 54:720–8

MacFarlane E, Benke G, Del Monaco A et al (2009) Cancer incidence and mortality in a historical cohort of Australian pest control workers. Occup Environ Med 66:818–823

Maddodi N, Setaluri V (2008) Role of UV in cutaneous melanoma. Photochem Photobiol 84(2): 528–36

Mahajan R, Blair A, Cable J et al (2007) Carbaryl exposure and incident cancer in the Agricultural Health Study. Int J Cancer 121:1799–1805

Meyskens FL, Farmer P, Fruehauf JP (2001a) Invited Review: redox regulation in human melanocytes and melanoma. Pigment Cell Res 14:148–154

Meyskens FL, McNulty SE, Buckmeier JA (2001b) Aberrant redox regulation in human metastatic melanoma cells compared to normal melanocytes. Free Radical Biol Med 31:799–808

Meyskens FL, Farmer P, Anton-Culver H (2004) Etiologic pathogenesis of melanoma: a unifying hypothesis for the missing attributable risk. Clin Cancer Res 10:2581–2583

Meyskens FL, Berwick M (2008) UV or not UV: metals are the answer. Cancer Epidem Biomarkers Prev 7:268–270

Nichols L, Sorahan T (2005) Cancer incidence and cancer morbidity in a cohort of UK semi conductor workers (1970–2002). Occup Med 55:625–630

Nielsen H, Henriksen L, Olsen JH et al (1996) Malignant melanoma among lithographers. Scand J Work Environ Health 22:108–11

Nyren O, McLaughlin JK, Gridley G et al (1995) Cancer risk after hip-replacement with metal implants: a population based cohort study in Sweden. J Natl Cancer Inst 87:28–33

O'Brien TJ, Ceryak S, Patierno SR (2003) Complexities of chromium carcinogenesis: role of cellular response, repair and recovery mechanisms. Mutation Res 533:3–36
Omenn GS, Goodman GE, Thornquist MD et al (1996) Effects of a combination of beta carotene and vitamin A on lung cancer and cardiovascular disease. New Eng J Med 334:1150–1155
Onega T, Baron J, Mackenzie T (2006) Cancer after total joint arthroplasty: a meta-analysis. Cancer Epidem Biomarkers Prev 15:1532–1537
Papageorgious I, Yin Z, Ladon D et al (2007) Genotoxic effects of particles of surgical cobalt chrome alloy on human cells of different age in vitro. Mutation Res 619:45–58
Perez-Gomez B, Pollan M, Gustavsson P et al (2004) Cutaneous melanoma: hints from occupational risks by anatomic site in Swedish men. Occup Environ Med 61:117–26
Pleasance ED, Cheetham K, Stephens PJ et al (2010) A comprehensive catalogue of somatic mutations from a human cancer genome. Nature 463:191–197
Rhodes AR, Seki Y, Fitzpatrick TB et al (1988) Melanosomal alterations in dysplastic melanocytic nevi: a quantitative, ultrastructural investigation. Cancer 61:358–69
Ruder AM, Hein MJ, Nilsen N et al (2006) Mortality among workers exposed to PCBs in an electrical capacitor manufacturing plant in Indiana: an update. Environ Health Perspect 114:18–23
Salnikow K, Zhitkovich A (2008) Genetic and epigenetic mechanisms in metal acarcenogenesis: nickel, arsenic and chromium. Chem Res Toxicol 21:28–44
Sarna T, Hyde JS, Swartz HM et al (1976) Ion-exchange in melanin: an electron spin resonance study with lanthanide probes. Science 192: 1132–4
Simon JD, Peles D, Wakamatsu K et al (2009) Current challenges in understanding melanogenesis: bridging chemistry, biological control, morphology, and function. Pigment Cell Melanoma Res 22:563–79
Sinks T, Steele G, Smith AB et al (1992) Mortality among workers exposed to polychlorinated biphenyls. Am J Epidemiol 136:389–98
Skipor A, Campbell P, Patterson C et al (2002) Serum and urine metal levels in patients with metal-on-metal surface arthroplasty. Mater Sci Mat Med 13:1227–1234
Snow ET (1991) A possible role for chromium (111) in genotoxicity. Environ Health Perspect 92: 75–81
Sotomatsu A, Tanaka M, Hirai S et al (1994) Synthetic melanin and ferric ions promote superoxide anion-mediated lipid peroxidation. FEBS Lett 342:105–108
Svensson SP, Lindgren S, Powell W et al (2003) Melanin inhibits cytotoxic effects of doxorubicin and daunorubicin in MOLT 4 cells. Pigment Cell Res 16:351–354
Visuri TI, Pukkala F, Pulkkinen P et al (2006) Cancer incidence and causes of death among total hip replacement patients: a review based on Nordic cohorts with a special emphasis on metal-on-metal bearings. Proc Inst Mech Eng H 220: 399–407
Weinlich G, Eisendle K, Hassler E (2006) Metallothionein-overexpression as highly significant prognostic factor in melanoma: a prespective study on 1270 patients. Br J Cancer 94: 835–41
Wondrak GT (2007) Let the sun shine in: mechanisms and potential for therapeutics in skin photodamage. Curr Opin Investig Drugs 8: 390–400
World Health Organization (1996) Biological monitoring of chemical exposure in the workplace, vol 1, p 102 WHO/HPR/OCH96.1. WHO, Geneva
Yiakouvaki A, Al SJ, Qengei A et al (2006) Caged-iron chelators a novel approach towards protecting skin cells against UVA-induced necrotic cell death. J Invest Dermatol 126:2287–95
Young JL (2009) Memorandum for secretaries of the military departments: minimizing the use of hexvalent chromium (Cr6+). Acquisition technology and logistics, Department of Defense, USA

Hepatitis B Virus and Cancer Prevention

6

Mei-Hwei Chang

Abstract Prevention of chronic hepatitis B virus (HBV) infection can successfully reduce the incidence of liver cancer. It is the first example of cancer-preventive vaccine in human, which proves that prevention of the infection of an infectious agent can prevent its related cancer.

Chronic HBV infection can lead to chronic hepatitis, liver cirrhosis, and hepatocellular carcinoma (HCC). HCC is one of the five major cancers in the world population. Hepatitis B virus (HBV) is the most important etiologic agent of liver cancer globally, particularly in high-prevalence areas of liver cancer.

The world's first universal HBV vaccination program was launched in Taiwan in July 1984. It has provided evidences that the prevalence of HBV infection has been reduced remarkably to approximately one-tenth of the original prevalence. Furthermore, reduction of the HCC incidence in children aged 6–14 years have been demonstrated in the vaccinated birth cohorts. Recently, we have further provided evidence that the prevention of HCC by this HBV vaccine extends from childhood to early adulthood.

The risk of developing HCC for vaccinated cohorts was associated with incomplete HBV vaccination; prenatal maternal hepatitis B surface antigen (HBsAg) seropositivity; and prenatal maternal HBeAg seropositivity. Failure to prevent HCC results mostly from unsuccessful control of HBV infection by highly infectious mothers. Future strategies to increase the global coverage rate of HBV immunization and to interrupt mother-to- infant transmission may enhance the cancer prevention effect of HBV immunization.

M.-H. Chang
Department of Pediatrics and Hepatitis Research Center, National Taiwan University Hospital, No.7, Chung-Shan S. Road, Taipei, Taiwan
e-mail: changmh@ntu.edu.tw

6.1 Infection and Cancer

Cancer is a major threat of human health. It accounted for 7.4 million deaths (around 13% of all deaths) in 2004 (http://www.who.int/mediacentre/factsheets/fs297/en/ index.html). Lung, stomach, liver, colon, and breast cancer cause the most cancer deaths. Action on major risk factors of cancer, such as smoking, diet, and infections, can prevent approximately one-third of cancers. The close relationship between infection and cancer provides an opportunity for cancer control through blocking the transmission routes of these infectious agents, prevention of infection by vaccines, and

H.-J. Senn and F. Otto (eds.), *Clinical Cancer Prevention*,
Recent Results in Cancer Research 188, DOI: 10.1007/978-3-642-10858-7_6,

development of effective and safe anti-infectious drugs (Table 6.1).

It has been estimated that chronic infections with viruses, bacteria, and parasites contribute to 17.8% of the global burden of cancer (Parkin 2006). Chronic infection with prolonged inflammation and regeneration often proceeds its related cancer development in human (Martin and Gutkind 2009). Worldwide, human viruses, such as Epstein-Barr virus (EBV), hepatitis B virus (HBV), hepatitis C virus (HCV), human papilloma virus (HPV), human T-cell lymphotropic virus (HTLV-1), and Kaposi's associated sarcoma virus (KSHV) contribute to approximately 10–15% of the cancers worldwide. Infection of bacteria, such as *Helicobater pylori*, and cancer (MALTOMA or gastric cancer) has been highly associated. The 2005 Nobel Prize in Physiology or Medicine recognized the work that showed *H. pyloric* infection as an important cause of peptic ulcer disease, and gastric malignancy. Three helminth infections have been classified as group 1 carcinogens to humans, namely *Schistosoma haematobium*, which is associated with cancer of the urinary bladder, and the food-borne liver flukes *Clonorchis sinensis* and *Opisthorchis viverrini* associated with cholangiocarcinoma of the liver (Vennervald and Polman 2009). Prevention of infection will reduce the risk of its related cancer development later in life.

The major mechanisms by which infectious agents can promote and maintain tumor formation includes persistent infection and chronic inflammation, virus-induced transformation with or without integration of viral genome into the host genome, and chronic suppression of the immune system by the infectious agent, such as the immunodeficiency (AIDS) caused by HIV infection (Dalton-Griffin and Kellam 2009).

Although an infectious agent may be recognized as the primary cause of cancer, it is a "necessary but insufficient cause." It suggests that while the infection is the primary cause, additional factors must be present to produce cancer. The most important contributing factor is the long-standing acute and chronic inflammation that results in marked changes in tissue structure and function (Graham and Asaka 2010).

Table 6.1 Infectious agents associated with cancer in human

Infectious agent	Associated cancer	Vaccine
Virus		
Epstein-Barr virus	Lymphoma, nasopharyngeal carcinoma	Nil
Hepatitis B virus	Hepatocellular carcinoma	Available
Hepatitis C virus	Hepatocellular carcinoma	Nil
Human papilloma virus	Cervical cancer, penis cancer	Available
Human T-cell lymphotropic virus	Adult T-cell leukemia	Nil
Kaposi's associated sarcoma virus	Kaposi's sarcoma	Nil
Bacteria		
Helicobater pylori	Gastric cancer/MALToma	Nil
Helminth		
Schistosoma haematobium	Urinary bladder cancer	Nil
Clonorchis sinensis	Cholangiocarcinoma	Nil
Opisthorchis viverrini	Cholangiocarcinoma	Nil

MALToma = mucosa-associated lymphoid tissue lymphomas

6.2 Disease Burden of Liver Cancer

Hepatocellular carcinoma (HCC) is one of the five main types of cancer leading to overall cancer mortality in human (http://www.who.int/mediacentre/factsheets/fs297/en/index.html). The majority of cases of HCCs occur in Asia and sub-Saharan Africa where the major risk factors are chronic infection with hepatitis B or C virus (HBV or HCV) (Wild and Montesano 2009). Although the majority of HCC cases occur in developing countries of Asia and Africa, the prevalence of liver cancer has risen considerably in Japan, Western Europe, as well as the United States. The occurrence of HCC in the United States has dramatically increased by more than 70% over the last 25 years (El-Serag 2004; Bishayee et al. 2010).

6.3 Hepatitis B Virus Infection and Hepatocellular Carcinoma

HCC most commonly develops in patients with chronic liver disease, the etiology of which includes viral hepatitis (B and C), alcohol, obesity, iron overload, and dietary carcinogens, including aflatoxins and nitrosamines (Bishayee et al. 2010). Among them, chronic HBV is the most important etiologic agent of HCC in the world population, particularly in high-prevalence areas of liver cancer (Beasley 2009).

HBV infection causes 60–80% of the HCC globally. Annually, approximately 340,000 chronic HBV infection-related liver cancer deaths occur; HBV is the most common cause of infection-related cancer deaths (http://www.who.int/en/). Chronic HBV infection can lead to chronic hepatitis, liver cirrhosis, and liver cancer.

In endemic areas of HBV infection, most chronic hepatitis B surface antigen (HBsAg) carriers were infected before 2 years of age. In parts of Africa, such as rural Senegal, horizontal infection occurs in very early childhood. By the age of 2 years, 25% of children were infected, while at age 15, the infection rate was 80% (Feret et al. 1987). In most parts of Asia, the HBsAg carrier rate in the general population is approximately 5–20% (Chang 2000; Ganem and Prince 2004; Lavanchy 2004). In highly prevalent areas such as Taiwan, primary HBV infections occur mainly during infancy and early childhood (Hsu et al 1986). The hepatitis B surface antigen (HBsAg) seropositive rate remains stationary after the age of 2 years before the era of universal HBV vaccination.

The age and source of primary infection are important factors affecting the outcome. Mother-to-infant transmission is the major source of chronic HBV infection (approximately 40–50%) in Asia. Maternal serum HBsAg and HBeAg status affect the outcome of HBV infection in their offsprings. Before the era of HBV immunization program, around 90% of the infants of the hepatitis B e antigen (HBeAg) seropositive carrier mothers became HBsAg carriers (Stevens et al 1975). Worldwide, mothers are the driving force behind the infections that lead to HCC, because the HBV carrier state is inversely proportional to the age of infection. (Beasley 2009). In contrast, infants of HBeAg-negative HBsAg carrier mothers tend to develop acute or fulminant hepatitis B, <5% have chronic infection or remain uninfected (Chang et al 1987; Shiraki et al 1980).

Persistent viral replication with elevated serum HBV DNA level (>10,000 copies/mL) is a strong risk predictor of HCC. A prospective cohort study of 3,653 participants (aged 30–65 years) with chronic HBV infection in Taiwan revealed that the incidence of HCC increased with serum HBV DNA level at study entry in a dose–response relationship ranging from 108 per 100,000 person-years for an HBV DNA level of <300 copies/mL to 1,152 per 100,000 person-years for an HBV DNA level of ≥1 million

6

copies/mL. Participants with persistent elevation of serum HBV DNA level during follow-up had the highest hepatocellular carcinoma risk (Chen et al. 2006). In addition, those infected chronically by HBV genotype C have a higher incidence rate of developing HCC than those infected by HBV genotype B (Yang et al. 2008).

6.4 Cancer Prevention Against Hepatocellular Carcinoma

HCC is one of the most common causes of cancer death worldwide. It has a poor prognosis in most occasions and a high recurrence rate after therapy. Therefore, prevention is more effective than therapy. Cancer prevention strategies against HCC can be divided into three levels: primary, secondary, and tertiary cancer prevention (Fig. 6.1).

Primary prevention: for general population.

1. Universal hepatitis virus vaccination is the most effective way to control HCC. Hepatitis B vaccine has been available for more than 25 years. Hepatitis C vaccine is still under investigation.
2. Screening the blood products, and proper sterilization of injection needles and syringes block the horizontal transmission of hepatitis virus.
3. Avoidance of risky behaviors may block HBV or HCV horizontal transmission.

Secondary prevention: for those with chronic HBV or HCV infection.

1. Antiviral therapy using interferon or nucleoside analogue against HBV to eliminate or reduce viral load may reduce liver injury, fibrosis, and the development of HCC in those who persistently respond to therapy. The supporting evidence for the prevention of HCC is much weaker than that of HBV vaccination (Lim et al. 2009). Continuous treatment with lamivudine delays clinical progression in patients with chronic hepatitis B and advanced fibrosis or cirrhosis by significantly reducing the incidence of hepatic decompensation and the risk of HCC. After a median duration of lamivudine treatment of 32.4 months, less HCC (3.9%) occurred in the lamivudine group than in the placebo group (7.4%) ($p = 0.047$) (Liaw et al. 2004). The main problem after long-term lamivudine therapy is drug resistance. The effect of HCC prevention using newer nucleoside/nucleotide analogues with lower drug resistance rate remains to be elucidated.

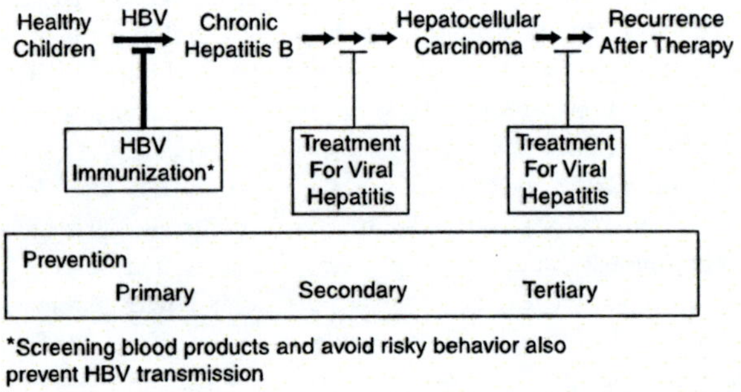

Fig. 6.1 Strategies to prevent viral hepatitis-associated hepatocellular carcinoma (HCC). The most effective way is primary prevention by immunization to prevent oncogenic hepatitis virus infection. Secondary prevention strategies are directed on reducing the complication and HCC rates in those with chronic viral hepatitis. Tertiary prevention strategy is to prevent late recurrence of HCC

2. Avoidance of aflatoxin exposure, metabolic syndrome, and other risky behaviors or environmental factors (Wild and Montesano 2009).

Tertiary prevention: for HCC patients who have been treated successfully by surgery, liver transplantation, or local therapy to prevent late tumor recurrence.

1. Antiviral therapy against HBV or HCV may potentially prevent late tumor recurrence (Breitenstein et al 2009).

Although in its infancy, several phytochemicals such as oltipraz, chlorophyllin, and resveratrol show promise as potential candidates for chemoprevention of hepatocarcinogenesis and as adjunctive chemotherapeutic agents in the treatment of HCC (Bishayee et al. 2010; Kensler et al 2004; Mann et al 2009). Among the above-mentioned strategies of cancer prevention, universal vaccination to block both mother-to-infant and horizontal transmission routes of HBV infection is proved to be the most effective and safe one.

6.5 Hepatitis B Vaccination Program

Passive immunization using hepatitis B immunoglobulin (HBIG) provides temporary immunity with higher cost, while active immunization using HBV vaccines provides long-term immunity and protection with lower expense.

Globally strategies for the hepatitis B vaccination in infancy can be divided into three main strategies depending on both the budget of the government for HBV immunization and the prevalence rate of HBsAg carriage. It is very important for a successful universal vaccination program to cover the expense of the vaccines and/or HBIG. In developing countries or countries with low prevalence of HBV infection and limited resources, immunization with three doses of HBV vaccine in a 0-, 1-, and 6-month schedule without antenatal screening of the maternal HBV markers and administration of HBIG is an effective and economic way for HBV infection and hepatoma control. Such programs have been successful in Thailand and many other countries in Asia (Poovorawan et al 2000).

In countries with high prevalence of HBV infection, screening of maternal HBsAg and HBeAg is conducted during pregnancy. In addition to active immunization with three or four doses of HBV vaccines, passive immunization with a dose of HBIG is given to the neonates within 24 h after birth to neutralize HBV transmitted from the mother during perinatal period. The world's first universal hepatitis B vaccination program was launched in July 1984 in Taiwan (Chen et al. 1987). The expense for all the vaccines and HBIG given to the infants were covered by the government. In all, the coverage rate of three-dose hepatitis B vaccine for neonates was around 84–94%.

In developed countries such as United States, pregnant women were screened for serum HBsAg but not HBeAg. In addition to three doses of HBV vaccine to every infants, all infants of HBsAg-positive mothers received HBIG within 24 h after birth (Shepard et al. 2006). This strategy saves the cost of maternal HBeAg screening, but increases the cost of HBIG, which is much more costlier than vaccine.

6.6 Effective Reduction of Chronic HBV Infection by Universal Hepatitis B Immunization

HBV vaccine has been part of the WHO global immunization resulting in major declines in acute and chronic HBV infection (Beasley 2009). Approximately 90–95% the incidence of chronic HBV infection in children has been reduced remarkably in areas where universal HBV vaccination in infancy has been successfully introduced.

6

Serial epidemiologic surveys of HBV markers were conducted before and 5, 10, 15, and 20 years after the implementation of the vaccination program in Taiwan (Hsu et al 1986; Tsen et al. 1991; Chen et al. 1996; Ni et al. 2001, 2007). The HBsAg carrier rate decreased significantly from around 10% before the vaccination program to 0.6–0.7% afterward in vaccinated children younger than 20 years of age. The total infection rate (anti-HBc seropositive rate) declined from 38% to 16% and further down to 4.6% in children 15–20 years after the program (Ni et al. 2007). Similar effect has also been observed in many other countries (Whittle et al. 1995; Jang et al. 2001), where universal vaccination programs have been successfully conducted. Universal HBV vaccination in infancy is more effective than selective immunization for high-risk groups.

The causes of breakthrough HBV infection in vaccinees include high maternal viral load (Lee et al 1986), intrauterine infection (Tang et al. 1998; Lin et al 1987), surface gene mutants (Hsu et al 1999; 2004; 2010), genetic hyporesponsiveness, and immune compromised host.

6.7 The Effect on Liver Cancer Prevention by Vaccination

In most countries, the age of peak incidence for HCC is after 40 years. Theoretically, it will take at least 40 years to see the effect of HCC prevention by HBV vaccination program in infancy. HCC in children is closely related to HBV infection. Previous studies in Taiwan revealed that the characteristics of childhood HCC are similar to that in adults (Chang et al. 1989). It is therefore plausible to study the effect of HBV vaccination on the prevalence of childhood HCC, in order to facilitate the understanding of the possible effect of liver cancer prevention by HBV vaccination.

In comparison to most other parts of the world, Taiwan has a high prevalence of HBV infection and HCC in children. Children with HCC in Taiwan are nearly 100% HBsAg seropositive, 86% of them are HBeAg negative, and their mothers are mostly (94%) HBsAg seropositive (Chang et al. 1989). The histologic features of HCC are similar to that in adult HCC. Most (80%) of the nontumor liver tissues have liver cirrhosis. Integration of HBV genome into host genome was demonstrated in the childhood HCC tissues (Chang et al. 1991).

Prevention of chronic HBV infection by immunization can successfully reduce the incidence of liver cancer (Table 6.2). Universal hepatitis B vaccination program has had a remarkable effect on the reduction of HCC incidence in children. The annual incidence of HCC in Taiwanese children aged 6–14 years was reduced from 0.52–0.54 per 100,000 children born before July 1984 to 0.13–0.20 per 100,000 children born after the vaccination program (Chang et al 1997, 2000). The cancer prevention effect by the universal HBV vaccine program has extended further beyond childhood after 20 years of the program (Table 6.2). HCC incidence was statistically significantly lower among children and adolescents aged 6–19 years in vaccinated compared with unvaccinated birth cohorts,

Table 6.2 The effect of HBV vaccination on HCC prevention in children and adolescents in Taiwan (Chang et al 1997, 2000, 2005, 2009)

Age group (Years)	HBV vaccinated Birth cohort	HCC incidence Rate (per 10^5)	RR
6–9	No	0.492	1 (referent)
	Yes	0.152	0.31
10–14	No	0.562	1 (referent)
	Yes	0.194	0.35
15–19	No	0.598	1 (referent)
	Yes	0.158	0.26
Total 6–19	No	0.565	1 (referent)
	Yes	0.169	0.30

RR = risk ratio

with a relative risk of 0.30. Studies in Thailand also showed declines in HCC incidence as a result of at-birth HBV immunization programs (Wichajarn et al 2008).

6.8 Problems and Strategies of Successful HCC Prevention by Hepatitis B Vaccination

Universal vaccination in infancy is most cost-effective toward a successful control of HBV-related HCC. WHO adopts HBV as the seventh immunogen in the EPI, its global infant immunization program. In spite of the great success in reduction of HCC incidence in children and adolescents, there is still approximately one-third of HCC not prevented by the universal HBV vaccination program. Better understanding of the causes of HCC prevention failure will be the key to design better strategies for HCC eradication. Current data revealed that HCC prevention failure is significantly associated with incomplete HBV vaccination/inadequate resources, and breakthrough HBV infection (Chang et al 2005, 2009).

Further increase of the global coverage rates of infant HBV vaccination is an important issue toward a better HCC control. Coverage of the expense of HBV vaccines in developing countries by the government or a vaccine fund is of vital important to effectively enhance the HBV vaccine coverage rate. It is particularly urgent in areas where HBV infection and HCC are prevalent. Up to 2008, according to the report from WHO, a total of approximately 71% (177 countries) have followed the WHO recommendation of HBV vaccination in infancy, with a coverage rate of >80% for three doses of HBV vaccine in 138 countries (WHO 2010).

In spite of enormous achievement made before, recent progress in many countries, including the developed countries, has been slow (Beasley 2009). Efforts to further increase the coverage rates of HBV vaccines globally should be actively made. In some developed countries, due to the competition of other new vaccines, HBV has not captured sufficient attention from the government (Van Herck et al. 2008). It is of vital importance to convince the government of the countries without a universal HBV vaccination program to establish a program and to encourage the countries with low coverage rate to increase the rates.

Failure to prevent HCC results mostly from unsuccessful control of HBV infection by highly infectious mothers. Approximately 90% of the mothers of the HCC children with known serum HBsAg status were positive for HBsAg (Chang et al 2009). This provides evidence to support that maternal transmission is the main route of HBV transmission in HCC children who failed to be protected by HBV immunization (Chang et al 2005). The risk of developing HCC for vaccinated cohorts was statistically significantly associated with prenatal maternal HBsAg seropositivity and HBeAg seropositivity. Future strategies to interrupt mother-to- infant transmission may enhance the cancer prevention effect of HBV immunization.

Infants of HBsAg carrier mothers with positive HBeAg and/or high viral load are the high-risk group of breakthrough HBV infection, in spite of immunoprophy-laxis with combination of passive (HBIG) and active (vaccine) immunization. Preliminary clinical trials using nucleoside analogue during last trimester of pregnancy to prevent mother-to-infant transmission have been conducted (Van Zonneveld et al. 2003; Xu et al. 2009). Yet the efficacy and safety need further evaluation.

6.9 Implications and Future Prospects

Hepatitis B vaccine has been proved to be safe, cheap, and highly immunogenic, with long-term efficacy. Universal HBV vaccination starting from the first day of life is the most important way to prevent HBV-related HCC. Successful

6

prevention of chronic hepatitis B virus (HBV) infection can reduce the incidence of liver cancer. It is the first example of cancer-preventive vaccine in human, which proves that prevention of the infection of an oncogenic infectious agent can prevent its related cancer.

To achieve a better effect of primary prevention against HCC, a higher global coverage rates of HBV vaccination in early infancy and better strategies against breakthrough HBV infection are needed.

The concept of a cancer-preventive vaccine, using HBV as the first example, can be applied to other infectious agents and their related cancers. Human papillomavirus (HPV) is responsible for 99.7% of cervical cancer patients and an estimated 5% of all cancers worldwide. Safe and effective virus-like- particle-derived prophylactic HPV vaccines are available to most nations (Moscicki 2008). HPV vaccination to prevent cervical cancer and other HPV-associated diseases will become the second example of cancer-preventive vaccine in human. However, strategies to reduce the very high cost of the current HPV vaccines are needed to make it available for most developing nations with high incidences of cervical cancer. Other cancer vaccines against oncogenic microorganisms such as HCV, EB virus, *H. pylori*, etc. are still under investigation.

Acknowledgment National Health Research Institutes, Taiwan (NHRI-EX94- 9418BI, NHRIEX95-9418BI,NHRI-EX96-9418BI,NHRI-EX97-9418BI, NHRI-EX98-9418BI, NHRIEX99-9418BI).

References

Beasley RP (2009) Rocks along the road to the control of HBV and HCC. Ann Epidemiol 19:231–234

Bishayee A, Politis T, Darvesh AS (2010) Resveratrol in the chemoprevention and treatment of hepatocellular carcinoma. Cancer Treat Rev 36:43–53

Breitenstein S, Dimitroulis D, Petrowsky H, Puhan MA, Müllhaupt B, Clavien PA (2009) Systematic review and meta-analysis of interferon after curative treatment of hepatocellular carcinoma in patients with viral hepatitis. Br J Surg 96:975–981

Chang MH, Lee CY, Chen DS, Hsu HC, Lai MY (1987) Fulminant Hepatitis in children in Taiwan: the important role of hepatitis B virus. J Pediatr 111:34–39

Chang MH, Chen DS, Hsu HC, Hsu HY, Lee CY (1989) Maternal transmission of hepatitis B virus in childhood hepatocellular carcinoma. Cancer 64:2377–2380

Chang MH, Chen PJ, Chen JY et al (1991) Hepatitis B virus integration in hepatitis B virus related hepatocellular carcinoma in Childhood. Hepatology 13:316–20

Chang MH, Chen CJ, Lai MS et al (1997) Universal hepatitis B vaccination in Taiwan and the incidence of hepatocellular carcinoma in children. N Engl J Med 336:1855–1859

Chang MH, Shau WY, Chen CJ et al (2000) The effect of universal hepatitis B vaccination on hepatocellular carcinoma rates in boys and girls. JAMA 284:3040–42

Chang MH (2000) Prospects for hepatitis B virus eradication and control of hepatocellular carcinoma. Bailliere's Clin Gastroenterol 13:511–517

Chang MH, Chen TH, Hsu HM et al (2005) Prevention of heaptocellular carcinoma by universal vaccination against hepatitis B virus: the effect and problems. Clin Cancer Res 11:7953–7957

Chang MH, You SL, Chen CJ et al (2009) Decreased incidence of hepatocellular carcinoma in hepatitis B vaccinees: a 20-year follow-up study. J Natl Cancer Inst 101:1348–1355

Chen CJ, Yang H-I, Su J et al; for the REVEAL-HBV Study Group (2006) Risk of hepatocellular carcinoma across a biological gradient of serum hepatitis B virus DNA level. JAMA 295:65–73

Chen DS, Hsu NH, Sung JL et al (1987) A mass vaccination program in Taiwan against hepatitis B virus infection in infants of hepatitis B surface antigen-carrier mothers. JAMA 257:2597–603

Chen HL, Chang MH, Ni YH et al (1996) Seroepidemiology of hepatitis B virus infection in children - ten years of mass vaccination in Taiwan. J Am Med Assoc 276:906–908

Dalton-Griffin L, Kellam P (2009) Infectious causes of cancer and their detection. J Biol 8:67.1–67.5

El-Serag HB (2004) Hepatocellular carcinoma: recent trends in the United States. Gastroenterology 127:S27–34

Graham DY, Asaka M (2010) Eradication of gastric cancer and more efficient gastric cancer surveillance in Japan: two peas in a pod. J Gastroenterol 45:1–8

Feret E, Larouze B, Dip B, Sow M, London WT, Blumberg BS (1987) Epidemiology of hepatitis B virus infection in the rural community of Tip, Senegal. Am J Epidemiol 125:140–9

Ganem D, Prince AM (2004) Hepatitis B virus infection natural history and clinical consequences. N Engl J Med 350:1118–1129

Hsu HY, Chang MH, Chen DS, Lee CY, Sung JL (1986) Baseline seroepidemiology of hepatitis B virus infection in children in Taipei, 1984: a study just before mass hepatitis B vaccination program in Taiwan. J Med Virol 18:301–307

Hsu HY, Chang MH, Liaw SH, Ni YH, Chen HL (1999) Changes of hepatitis B surface variants in carrier children before and after universal vaccination in Taiwan. Hepatology 30:1312–1317

Hsu HY, Chang MH, Ni YH, Chen HL (2004) Survey of hepatitis B surface variant infection in children 15 years after nationwide vaccination program in Taiwan. Gut 53:1499–1503

Hsu HY, Chang MH, Ni YH, et al (2010) No increase of hepatitis B surface antigen mutant prevailing in a children and adolescent population fully covered by universal infant immunization. J Infect Dis 2010; 201:1192–200.

Jang MK, Lee JY, Lee JH, Kim YB, Kim HY, Lee MS, Park CK, Yoo JY (2001) Seroepidemiology of HBV infection in South Korea, 1995 through 1999. Korean J Intern Med 16:153–159

Kensler TW, Egner PA, Wang JB et al (2004) Chemoprevention of hepatocellular carcinoma in aflatoxin endemic areas. Gastroenterology 127(Suppl 1):S310–318

Lavanchy D (2004) Hepatitis B virus epidemiology, disease burden, treatment, and current and emerging prevention and control measures. J Viral Hepat 11:97–107

Lee SD, Lo KJ, Wu JC et al (1986) (1986) Prevention of maternal-infant hepatitis B virus transmission by immunization: the role of serum hepatitis B virus DNA. Hepatology 6:369–373

Liaw Y-F, Sung JJY, Chow WC et al (2004) Lamivudine for patients with chronic hepatitis B and advanced liver disease. N Engl J Med 351:1521–1531

Lim SG, Mohammed R, Yuen MF, Kao JH (2009) Prevention of hepatocellular carcinoma in hepatitis B virus infection. J Gastroenterol Hepatol 24:1352–1357

Lin HH, Lee TY, Chen DS et al (1987) Transplacental leakage of HBeAg-positive maternal blood as the most likely route in causing intrauterine infection with hepatitis B virus. J Pediatr 111:877–881

Mann CD, Neal CP, Garcea G, Manson MM, Dennison AR, Berry DP (2009) Phytochemicals as potential chemopreventive and chemotherapeutic agents in hepatocarcinogenesis. Eur J Cancer Prev 18:13–25

Martin D, Gutkind JS (2009) Human tumor- associated viruses and new insights into the molecular mechanisms of cancer. Oncogene 27:S31–S42

Moscicki AB (2008) HPV vaccines: today and in the future. J Adolesc Health 43:S26–S40

Ni YH, Chang MH, Huang LM et al (2001) Hepatitis B virus infection in children and adolescents in a hyperendemic area: 15 years after mass hepatitis B vaccination. Ann Intern Med 135:796–800

Ni YH, Huang LM, Chang MH et al (2007) Two decades of universal hepatitis B vaccination in Taiwan: impact and implication for future strategies. Gastroenterology 132:1287–1293

Parkin DM (2006) The global health burden of infection-associated cancers in the year 2002. Int J Cancer 118:3030–3044

Poovorawan Y, Theamboonlers A, Vimolket T et al (2000) Impact of hepatitis B immunization as part of the EPI. Vaccine 19:943–949

Shepard CW, Simard EP, Finelli L, Fiore AF, Bell BP (2006) Hepatitis B virus infection: epidemiology and vaccination. Epidemiol Rev 28:112–125

Shiraki K, Yoshihara N, Sakurai M, Eto T, Kawana T (1980) Acute hepatitis B in infants born to carrier mother with the antibody to hepatitis B e antigen. J Pediatr 97:768–70

Stevens CE, Beasley RP, Tsui J, Lee WC (1975) Vertical transmission of hepatitis B antigen in Taiwan. N Engl J Med 292:771–4

Vennervald BJ, Polman K (2009) Helminths and malignancy. Parasite Immunol 31:686–96

Tang JR, Hsu HY, Lin HH, Ni YH, Chang MH (1998) Hepatitis B surface antigenemia at birth: a long-term follow-up study. J Pediatr 133:374–377

Tsen YJ, Chang MH, Hsu HY, Lee CY, Sung JL, Chen DS (1991) Seroepidemiology of hepatitis B virus infection in Taipei, 1989- Five years after a mass hepatitis B vaccination program. J Med Virol 34:96–99

6

Van Herck K, Vorsters A, Van Damme P (2008) Prevention of viral hepatitis (B and C) reassessed. Best Pract Res Clin Gastroenterol 22:1009–1029

Van Zonneveld M, van Nunen AB, Niesters HGM, de Man RA, Schalm SW, Janssen HLA (2003) Lamivudine treatment during pregnancy to prevent perinatal transmission of hepatitis B virus infection. J Viral Hepat 10:294–297

Whittle HC, Maine N, Pilkington J et al (1995) Long-term efficacy of continuing hepatitis B vaccination in infancy in two Gambian villages. Lancet 29(345):1089–1092

WHO (2010) Report on the Expanded Program on Immunization (EPI) of the World Health Organisation (WHO) Department of Vaccines and Biologicals (Post-exposure immunization for hepatitis B). WHO, Geneva. www.who.immunization/

Wichajarn K, Kosalaraksa P, Wiangnon S (2008) Incidence of hepatocellular carcinoma in children in Khon Kaen before and after national hepatitis B vaccine program. Asian Pac J Cancer Prev 9:507–9

Wild CP, Montesano R (2009) A model of interaction: aflatoxins and hepatitis viruses in liver cancer aetiology and prevention. Cancer Lett 286:22–28

Xu WM, Cui YT, Wang L et al (2009) Efficacy and safety of lamivudine in late pregnancy for the prevention of mother-child transmission of hepatitis B: a multicentre, randomized, double-blind, placebo-controlled study. J Viral Hepat 16:94–103

Yang HI, Yeh SH, Chen PJ et al (2008) Associations between hepatitis B virus genotype and mutants and the risk of hepatocellular carcinoma. J Natl Cancer Inst 100:1134–1143

Chemoprevention of Hepatocellular Carcinoma in Chronic Hepatitis C

7

Timothy R. Morgan

Abstract Hepatitis C virus (HCV) infection causes chronic hepatitis, which can progress to cirrhosis and hepatocellular carcinoma (HCC). The incidence of hepatocellular carcinoma in the United States tripled between 1975 and 2005, and is expected to increase further, and to remain elevated for more than 20 years. Curing hepatitis C infection in patients with cirrhosis through treatment with peginterferon and ribavirin reduces the risk of developing hepatocellular carcinoma. Several noncurative treatments also appear to reduce the risk of hepatocellular carcinoma in patients with chronic hepatitis C. Prospective studies report a reduced incidence of hepatocellular carcinoma among patients treated with a mixture of carotenoids with or without myo-inositol, with vitamin K_2, or with polyprenoic acid (an acyclic retinoid). Uncontrolled and/or retrospective studies have reported beneficial effects of treatment with Sho-saiko-to, glycyrrhizin and ursodeoxycholic acid on hepatocellular carcinoma incidence. Meta-analyses of epidemiologic studies show a reduced risk of hepatocellular carcinoma among liver disease patients who drink two or more cups of coffee per day. Numerous agents prevent or reduce hepatocarcinogenesis in animal models. An ongoing Phase II clinical trial is evaluating *S*-adenosylmethionine (SAMe) as a potential chemopreventive agent in hepatitis C cirrhosis. Overall, these data suggest that chemoprevention of hepatocellular carcinoma in patients with chronic hepatitis C is an achievable objective.

Conflict of Interest: I receive support for clinical trials in hepatitis C treatment from Hoffmann-LaRoche, Schering Plough, Merck and Vertex. Within the past 2 years, I have served on the Advisory Board, Speaker's Bureau, or have been a consultant for Hoffmann-LaRoche, Vertex, and/or Gilead.

7.1 Hepatitis C

The existence of a hepatitis C virus (HCV) was suspected in 1975 when investigators found cases of hepatitis in transfusion recipients, which were not caused by infection with hepatitis A or hepatitis B virus (Feinstone et al. 1975). Posttransfusion non-A, non-B hepatitis, as the disease was called for many years, caused minimally symptomatic

T.R. Morgan
Gastroenterology Section VA Long Beach Healthcare System,
5901 E. Seventh Street – 11, Long Beach, CA 90822, USA and

University of California, Irvine, CA, USA
e-mail: timothy.morgan@va.gov

H.-J. Senn and F. Otto (eds.), *Clinical Cancer Prevention*,
Recent Results in Cancer Research 188, DOI: 10.1007/978-3-642-10858-7_7,

7

acute disease (rarely with jaundice) with relatively mild histological injury (Seeff 2009). Initially described in patients who had received blood transfusions, non-A, non-B hepatitis was subsequently reported in community-acquired settings. In 1989, the hepatitis C virus was discovered by using molecular biological techniques to probe an expression library made from the serum of a patient with chronic, posttransfusion non-A, non-B hepatitis (Choo et al. 1989). Discovery of the hepatitis C virus led to development of sensitive serum assays for the presence of hepatitis C antibody (Kuo et al. 1989), and subsequently, to the perfection of assays to detect HCV RNA in the serum.

The epidemiology and natural history of hepatitis C infection has been studied for many years. HCV is spread by percutaneous routes. In the United States, intravenous drug use is the most common source of infection while blood transfusions account for approximately 10% of infections. In other countries, hepatitis C is reported to have been spread iatrogenically through the use of contaminated needles or transfusion of contaminated blood (Bosch et al. 2005). Hepatitis C is found in healthy blood donors throughout the world. In the United States, central Europe, China, and Australia, less than 1% of blood donors are infected with hepatitis C; rates of 1–5% are reported in healthy blood donors in countries in the former Soviet Union and in several Middle Eastern countries. Approximately 85% of patients who are acutely infected with hepatitis C become chronically infected. The natural history of patients who are chronically infected is variable. A minority have minimal or no fibrosis despite decades of infection However, most patients with chronic hepatitis C infection have progressive liver fibrosis, although the rate of fibrosis progression is variable and cannot be predicted in an individual patient. Hepatitis C is a common cause of cirrhosis throughout the world.

Hepatitis C can be cured by treatment with interferon and ribavirin. Initial studies from 1989, using interferon monotherapy for 24 weeks, reported a response rate of approximately 5% (Davis et al. 1989). However, multiple advances during the 1990s, using longer treatment periods (48 weeks), development of pegylated (long-acting) interferon, and the addition of a second antiviral agent (ribavirin) resulted in improvement in the sustained virological response (SVR, cure) rate (in Phase III trials) to approximately 50% by 2002. The SVR rate in community-based studies is closer to 30–40% (Backus et al. 2007). Despite this remarkable achievement, side effects of peginterferon and ribavirin are common, and consequently approximately 75% of patients are not eligible for treatment. Overall, an estimated 5–10% of patients infected with hepatitis C can be cured through treatment with peginterferon and ribavirin.

7.2 Hepatocellular Carcinoma

Hepatocellular carcinoma is the fifth most common cancer in the world and the third most common cause of cancer-related mortality (Parkin 2001). Hepatitis C is a recognized cause of hepatocellular carcinoma. In 2002 in the United States, hepatitis C was estimated to be the underlying cause of HCC in approximately 27% of cases (El-Serag and Rudolph 2007), a number which, in the author's experience, markedly underestimates its true contribution to hepatocellular carcinoma. In Europe, hepatitis C causes 27–75% of HCC while in Japan it causes 80–90% of HCC (Blonski and Reddy 2008).

The incidence of hepatocellular carcinoma in the United States increased threefold between 1975 and 2005 (Altekruse et al. 2009), and is expected to increase further in the next few years, and to remain significantly greater than the current rate for the next 20 years (Davis et al. 2010). Efforts to detect HCC at an early stage, through routine ultrasound examination of the liver, with or without alpha-fetoprotein testing, in patients with cirrhosis, has been recommended by the American Association for the Study of Liver Diseases (Bruix and Sherman 2005), European Association for Study of the Liver and Asian Pacific Association for the Study of the Liver. Although liver transplantation in patients with early hepatocellular carcinoma is curative, less than 10% of patients with HCC in the United States are eligible for liver transplantation (Bruix and Sherman 2005). Noncurative treatments included trans-arterial chemoemoblization (TACE, lipiodol, Yttrium spheres) of the tumor. Locally ablative treatments, such as radiofrequency ablation, microwave ablation, and percutaneous ethanol injection, reduce tumor burden, but are rarely curative. In the United States, 1-year survival rates have improved during the past 20 years, but remain close to 50% (Altekruse et al. 2009).

The poor response to treating established hepatocellular carcinoma has led to attempts to prevent its development. These treatments can be divided into those which are directed at curing the hepatitis C infection and those which are not curative. Within these divisions, there are prospective, randomized trials of moderate or high quality as well as nonrandomized, noncontrolled or retrospective studies of lesser significance. Finally, there are multiple studies in rodent models of chemical-induced carcinogenesis which appear promising and which will be summarized very briefly.

7.3 Prevention of Hepatocellular Carcinoma

7.3.1 Curative Treatment

In the late 1990s, several investigators in Japan, as well as those in Italy and Argentina, reported that patients treated with interferon were less likely to develop hepatocellular carcinoma. These findings were examined in greater detail in several recent investigations. The Italian Association for the Study of Liver Diseases retrospectively identified 920 patients with hepatitis C cirrhosis who had received treatment with interferon, of who 124 achieved SVR (Bruno et al. 2007). During a median follow-up of 8 years, the incidence rate of HCC was 0.66 (95% CI: 0.27–1.37) per 100 person-years of follow-up in those achieving SVR as compared with 2.10 (95% CI: 1.75–2.51) among subjects without SVR. By Kaplan-Meyer analysis, the incidences of HCC differed significantly between those with SVR and those who did not achieve SVR ($p < 0.01$ by log-rank test). A similar analysis was performed by investigators from Switzerland, Germany, the Netherlands, and Canada (Veldt et al. 2007). Among 479 patients with biopsy-proved cirrhosis (Ishak fibrosis score 4–6), 142 achieved SVR. Patients who achieved an SVR were followed for a median of 11 months while those not achieving SVR were followed for a median of 19 months. Achieving an SVR was associated with a significant reduction in the probability of developing liver failure (5-year occurrence: 0% in SVR versus 13.3% in non-SVR; $p < 0.001$). Achieving an SVR was associated with a nonsignificant reduction in the risk of developing hepatocellular carcinoma (5-year occurrence: 9.2% in SVR versus 13.1% in non-SVR; $p = 0.19$).

The Hepatitis C Antiviral Long-term Treatment of Cirrhosis (HALT-C) trial, an NIH-funded study of approximately 1,000 patients with hepatitis C and advanced fibrosis or cirrhosis, also evaluate the effect of achieving SVR on patients with chronic hepatitis C (Di Bisceglie et al. 2008). During a follow-up of 6 years, patients who achieved an SVR had an approximately 80% reduction in the development of hepatocellular carcinoma as compared with those who did not achieve SVR. These studies, taken as a whole, are consistent in finding that patients with hepatitis C and advanced fibrosis

7

or cirrhosis who achieve an SVR with interferon treatment have a significant reduction in the risk of developing hepatocellular carcinoma during the subsequent 5–8 years. However, of note, most studies report a small incidence of HCC in subjects who achieve SVR, suggesting that continued monitoring with ultrasound examination of the liver is warranted for many years after achieving SVR (Bruno et al. 2007; Veldt et al. 2007; George et al. 2009).

7.3.2 Treatments That Suppress Hepatitis C Virus

The primary objective of the HALT-C trial was to determine whether chronic treatment with peginterferon would reduce the incidence of decompensated liver disease and/or hepatocellular carcinoma in hepatitis C patients with advanced fibrosis or cirrhosis. Unfortunately, treatment for 3.5 years did not significantly reduce the development of either decompensated liver disease or hepatocellular carcinoma (Di Bisceglie et al. 2008; Lok et al. 2009). However, the major reason for failure to achieve a reduction in complications of liver disease might have been due to the relative lack of efficacy of the peginterferon, which resulted in an approximately 0.5 $\log_{10}$ reduction in HCV RNA (serum HCV RNA level of approximately $10^{6.5}$ IU/mL in control patients and $10^{6.0}$ IU/mL in patients receiving peginterferon). Subsequent analysis, comparing subjects in whom peginterferon treatment produced a >4 $\log_{10}$ reduction in HCV RNA with those in whom it produced a minimal reduction in HCV RNA (<1 $\log_{10}$), found that patients with marked reduction in HCV RNA had a significant reduction in subsequent development of decompensated liver disease (Shiffman et al. 2009). Thus, preliminary evidence suggests that treatment which effectively suppresses HCV RNA, even if it does not entirely clear the virus from the blood, may reduce the incidence of complications of liver disease. Further analyses of the HALT-C data for the effects of long-term peginterferon treatment on the incidence of HCC over a longer time period are in progress.

7.3.3 Noncurative Chemoprevention

In theory, noncurative treatments could be directed at preventing the progression of fibrosis (reducing the development of cirrhosis) or at counteracting potential carcinogenic pathways (e.g., oxidative stress, inflammation, COX-2, Wnt signaling). It is likely that several pathophysiologic mechanisms are common to both pathways. For example, oxidative stress and inflammation could contribute to fibrosis progression and carcinogenesis. Thus, treatments inhibiting these mechanisms may be beneficial by reducing either fibrosis, progression of carcinogenesis, or both pathways.

7.3.4 Prospective Randomized Trials: Carotenoids and Phytochemicals

Carotenoids are naturally occurring compounds found in fruits and vegetables (Nishino et al. 2009). More than 700 carotenoids have been described, of which approximately 40 are found in daily foods and approximately 20 have been detected in humans. Beta-carotene, which can be converted to vitamin A in the body, is the most extensively studied carotenoid. Other carotenoids include alpha-carotene, lutein, lycopene, and β-cryp-α-carotene. Carotenoids are important as antioxidants and, based on this mechanism of action, have been widely studied as chemopreventive agents. Several members of the carotenoid family may reduce the development of cancer in animal models. Studies of carotenoids and vitamin A as chemopreventive agents in human cancer are less clear (Bjelakovic et al. 2004).

Nishino and colleagues from Kyoto, Japan conducted a prospective study of a mixture of carotenoids in patients with viral hepatitis, 90% of whom had hepatitis C (Nishino 2007). A total of 46 patients were randomized to receive a pill containing 20 mg of carotenoids per day (lycopene 10 mg; β-carotene 6 mg; α-carotene 3 mg, other carotenoids 1 mg; packaged into a capsule containing α-tocopherol 50 mg). Patients in the control group ($n = 46$) received symptomatic treatment. Patients were followed for 2–5 years (median 3.4 years) for the development of HCC. After 4 years, patients receiving the carotenoids had a greater than 50% reduction in the incidence of HCC (34.6% versus 12.3%, $p < 0.02$).

Nishino subsequently found that patients with hepatocellular carcinoma had low serum levels of β-cryptoxanthin, and that addition of β-cryptoxanthin to the drinking water of C3H/He male mice (spontaneous liver cancer model) reduced the incidence of HCC by 93% (Nishino 2009). Similarly, addition of myo-inositol reduced the incidence of HCC in this mouse model by 90%. Based on these data, Nishino developed a juice drink from Japanese mandarin oranges, which contained 3 mg of β-cryptoxanthin and 1 g of myo-inositol. In an uncontrolled trial, he administered the carotenoid-containing pill (above) along with the orange juice containing β-cryptoxanthin and myo-inositol to 24 subjects with chronic hepatitis. During a follow-up of 2.5 years, one patient (4.2%) developed hepatocellular carcinoma (Nishino 2009). As compared with his prior trial, 22.2% of untreated patients developed HCC during the first 2.5 years after enrollment. Although this study was uncontrolled, it suggests that treatment with a combination of carotenoids and with juice containing β-cryptoxanthin and myo-inositol may significantly reduce the risk of developing HCC in patients with hepatitis C. Further studies with carotenoids and myo-inositol as chemopreventive agents in hepatitis C appear to be reasonable.

Vitamin K is a cofactor for the enzyme that converts glutamate residues into γ-carboxyglutamate. Vitamin K is required for the synthesis of coagulation proteins, including prothrombin and factors VII, IX, and X, protein C, and protein S. Vitamin K is a family of proteins, including the naturally occurring forms (vitamins K_1 and K_2) as well as the synthetic form (vitamin K_3). Both vitamins K_2 and K_3 inhibit growth of human cancer cell lines and suppress induction of differentiation in several human myeloid leukemia cell lines. In a case report, vitamin K_2 has been used to treat myelodysplastic syndrome (Takami et al. 1999).

Based on the potential of vitamin K to inhibit tumor cell growth, Habu and colleagues conducted a prospective, randomized trial of vitamin K_2 (45 mg/day) versus no treatment in 43 women with biopsy-proven cirrhosis (>90% due to chronic hepatitis C) (Habu et al. 2004; Tamori et al. 2007). During a follow-up period of up to 7 years, 2/21 (9.5%) of patients receiving vitamin K_2 developed HCC as compared with 9/19 (47.4%) of patients receiving no treatment ($p < 0.02$ by log-rank test). On multivariate analysis, adjusting for differences in age, ALT, albumin, bilirubin, platelet count, alpha fetoprotein (AFP), and interferon treatment, vitamin K_2 treatment reduced the risk of HCC by >85% (risk ratio 1.26 (95% CI: 0.016–0.992; $p = 0.049$). No patient receiving vitamin K_2 developed a significant adverse reaction or dropped out of the study. These promising results, using a drug which is inexpensive and readily available, need to be confirmed in large, prospective, placebo-controlled trials.

7.3.5 Secondary Chemoprevention of HCC

Vitamin A and its derivatives, collectively termed retinoids, have marked effects on cell growth and differentiation and have cancer-preventing effects in several animal models of cancer, including hepatocellular carcinoma. Because of these effects and relative low toxicity, vitamin A

7

has been studied as a chemopreventive agent in several types of cancer. Muto and colleagues created synthetic vitamin A compounds, including the acyclic retinoid, polyprenoic acid (20 carbon) (Kojima et al. 2004). This compound inhibits phosphorylation of retinoid X receptor alpha, thereby altering gene expression (Moriwaki et al. 2007; Shimizu et al. 2009). It has relatively low toxicity in animal and human studies (Muto et al. 1996). It reduced growth of human hepatoma cell lines and inhibited chemical-induced hepatocarcinogenesis in rats as well as spontaneous hepatocellular carcinoma in mice (Moriwaki et al. 2007).

Muto and coworkers undertook a multicenter, prospective, randomized, placebo-controlled trial of 600 mg of polyprenoic acid daily versus placebo in 89 patients who had received complete resection or complete obliteration of HCC by percutaneous ethanol injection (70% had hepatitis C cirrhosis) (Muto et al. 1996). Treatment with polyprenoic acid or placebo was daily for 12 months; patients were followed thereafter for the development of a second hepatocellular carcinoma. During a median follow-up of 38 months, a second HCC occurred in 12/44 (27%) of patients receiving polyprenoic acid and 22/45 (49%) of patients receiving placebo ($p = 0.04$). The results were more striking when comparing the number of patients who developed a second primary HCC (defined as an HCC occurring in a different liver segment (for PEI) or at least 2 cm from the initial HCC (for resected HCC). Among subjects receiving polyprenoic acid, 7/44 (16%) developed a second primary HCC as compared with 20/45 (44%) of patients receiving placebo ($p < 0.004$). Follow-up of these patients for 6 years demonstrated improved overall survival in patients receiving polyprenoic acid (estimated 6-year survival of 74%) as compared with placebo (estimated 6-year survival 46%, $p = 0.04$) (Muto et al. 1999). One patient receiving polyprenoic acid had headaches and stopped treatment; there were no toxic side effects typical of retinoids, such as dry skin, cheilitis, or conjunctivitis. Although this was an investigation of prevention of secondary HCC, the relative safety of the drug and probably low cost suggest that it could be evaluated for the primary prevention of HCC.

7.3.6 Nonrandomized, Uncontrolled and/or Retrospective Clinical Trials

Sho-saiko-to (SST, also TJ-9) is a traditional Chinese herbal medicine derived from seven species of medicinal plants (Hirayama et al. 1989). The concentration of the seven plants in Sho-saiko-to is regulated in Japan (Oka et al. 1995). SST is widely used in Japan to treat various chronic diseases, especially chronic hepatitis. Studies in humans, many with hepatitis B, reported an improvement in ALT and AST with 12 weeks of SST administration (Hirayama et al. 1989) while 8 weeks of treatment improved subjective symptoms of chronic liver disease. Animal studies have reported that SST protects rats from carbon tetrachloride injury.

Beginning in 1985, Oka and colleagues enrolled 260 patients with biopsy-proven cirrhosis from chronic liver disease to either no treatment (control group) or to treatment with TJ-9, 7.5 g orally/day (Oka et al. 1995). Patients were followed for 5 years. Retrospective testing of stored serum on 94 patients revealed hepatitis C in 81%. Hepatocellular carcinoma developed in 63/260 patients during follow-up. HCC occurred within 6 months of enrollment in six patients; these were withdrawn from analysis. Overall, 23% of patients receiving TJ-9 developed HCC as compared with 34% receiving no treatment ($p = 0.07$). When the patients with HBsAg were removed from the analysis, HCC occurred in 22% of patients receiving TJ-9 as compared with 39% receiving no treatment ($p = 0.024$). Furthermore, TJ-9 appeared to improve 5-year survival. When considering the entire patient population, survival was 75% among cirrhotics receiving TJ-9 as compared with 61% among those receiving no treatment ($p = 0.053$). When patients with hepatitis B were removed from the analysis, TJ-9 treatment was associated with a significantly improved 5-year survival (76% versus 60%; $p = 0.043$).

Glycyrrhizin (an aqueous extract of licorice root [*glycyrrhizae radix*]) is one of the seven ingredients in Sho-saiko-to, and has been used independently as a chemopreventive agent. The presumed mechanism of action is a protective effect on cell membranes, resulting in less inflammation. The preparation Stronger Neo-Minophagen C (SNMC) is an aqueous preparation of 0.2% glycyrrhizin, 0.1% cysteine, and 2% glycine dissolved in physiologic solution. It is administered intravenously (usually 100 mL). In a randomized, double-blind, controlled trial SNMC administration improved ALT in patients with chronic hepatitis (Arase et al. 1997). Improvement in ALT and liver histology were reported in other clinical trials.

Arase and colleagues performed a nonrandomized study of SNMC as compared with no treatment in 193 patients with biopsy-proven hepatitis C cirrhosis (Arase et al. 1997). Eighty-four patients received SNMC, 100 mL intravenously daily for 8 weeks followed by intravenous administration two to seven times per week for up to 16 years (median 10.1 years). The control group received symptomatic treatment (including other herbal medicines and/or vitamin K) for up to 16 years (median 9.2 years). During follow-up, ALT was normal in 35.7% of patients receiving SNMC as compared with 6.4% receiving no treatment ($p < 0.0001$). The cumulative incidence of HCC was significantly lower in subjects receiving SNMC as compared with those receiving no treatment (15-year HCC rate. 12% for SNMC versus 25% for no treatment; $p = 0.032$). On multivariate analysis, subjects not treated with SNMC had an odds ratio of 2.49 for development of HCC (95% CI: 1.01–6.12; $p = 0.044$). This study raises the possibility that glycyrrhizin may reduce the risk of hepatocellular carcinoma in patients with chronic hepatitis C. However, since glycyrrhizin must be administered intravenously several times per week on a long-term basis, it is unlikely to be widely used in clinical practice.

Tarao and coworkers studied Sho-saiko-to, SNMC, and ursodeoxycholic acid as chemopreventive agents against hepatocellular carcinoma in 102 patients with hepatitis C and Child A cirrhosis (Tarao et al. 2005). Patients were treated with SNMC (60–100 mL, intravenously, two to three times per week), Sho-saiko-to (7.5 g/day, orally) or UDCA (usually 300 mg/day, orally) in an attempt to reduce the ALT to less than 80 IU/mL. Initial treatment could be started with any one of the drugs. If a patient's ALT did not decline to less than 80 IU/mL a second agent was added. If the ALT did not decline to less than 80 IU/mL with two agents, then a third drug was added. Patients were followed for up to 5 years; the average duration of treatment with UDCA was 37 months. The analysis compared the incidence of HCC in patients who received UDCA versus subjects who did not receive UDCA. The 5-year incidence of HCC was 17.9% (10/56) among subjects receiving UDCA and 39.1% (18/46) among subjects not receiving UDCA ($p = 0.025$). Detailed analyses did not suggest that use of either Sho-saiko-to or SNMC differed between subjects who received UDCA and those who did not receive UDCA. On multivariate analysis, nonuse of UDCA was significantly associated with HCC (odds ratio 2.76 versus use of UDCA, $p < 0.05$). UDCA is a safe and commonly used drug in patients with liver disease and it seems reasonable to consider its use in chemopreventive studies in chronic hepatitis C.

7.3.7 Epidemiologic Studies

Coffee contains antioxidants such as chlorogenic acids, as well as diterpenes, cafestol, and kahweol that may inhibit enzymes involved in carcinogenic detoxification (Bravi et al. 2007; Larsson and Wolk 2007). Coffee, caffeine, and chlorogenic acids have an inhibitory effect on liver carcinogenesis in rodents (Tanaka et al. 1990). Studies in humans with liver disease have reported a beneficial effect of coffee consumption on ALT (La Vecchia 2005; Ruhl and Everhart 2005a, b), liver disease (Ruhl and Everhart 2005a, b), cirrhosis (La Vecchia 2005), and progression of fibrosis in patients with chronic hepatitis C (Freedman et al. 2009; Modi et al. 2010). Multiple observational studies from Japan and southern Europe have evaluated the association between coffee drinking and hepatocellular carcinoma. Meta-analyses of these studies found that coffee consumption was associated with an approximately 40% relative risk reduction for hepatocellular carcinoma per two to three cups of coffee per day as compared with non-coffee drinkers (Larsson and Wolk 2007; Bravi et al. 2009). Although the relative risk is significant, caution is warranted in the application of the findings to hepatocellular carcinoma chemoprevention. First, the studies are observational, from two areas of the world. Second, they might be confounded by the potential for patients with greater liver damage to drink less coffee (caffeine is eliminate from the body by the liver). Finally, they are based on self-report of coffee intake (dietary recall) and often include patients with multiple types of liver disease (e.g., hepatitis C, hepatitis B, alcohol). Nevertheless, the data are consistent, and coffee is a relatively safe and inexpensive treatment, which may hold potential benefit for prevention of hepatocellular carcinoma in chronic hepatitis C.

7.3.8 Drugs Used to Treat Hepatocellular Carcinoma

Several drugs have been used to treat hepatocellular carcinoma, and it is possible that these drugs, or analogs, might be useful to prevent it. The tyrosine kinase inhibitor, sorafenib, prolongs survival in patients with hepatocellular carcinoma and relatively preserved liver function (Child A or B) (Llovet et al. 2008). It is orally active, and has tolerable toxicity, which might be reduced by use of a lower dose than is used for treatment of hepatocellular carcinoma. The long-acting somatostatin analog, octreotide, has been evaluated in two prospective, randomized trials from Greece and Crete (Kouroumalis et al. 1998; Dimitroulopoulos et al. 2007). Patients with unresectable hepatocellular carcinoma from hepatitis C and B were included in the studies. Both studies reported significantly longer survival in patients receiving octreotide as compared with the control group (median survival of 4 months versus 13 months, and median survival of 49 weeks versus 28 weeks). Octreotide needs to be administered subcutaneously or intramuscularly, making it less desirable for long-term chemoprevention trials. Tamoxifen is an antiestrogen, which reduced liver tumors in an animal model of chemical carcinogenesis (Di Bisceglie et al. 2005). Manesis and colleagues from Athens randomized 85 patients with HCC to various combinations of treatment with the leuteinizing hormone releasing hormone analog, triptorelin, and the antiestrogen drugs, flutamide or tamoxifen (Manesis et al. 1995). They found that the tamoxifen group had a significantly longer survival (282 days) as compared with the flutamide (128 days) or placebo group (127 days). In multivariate analysis, tamoxifen treatment was independently associated with improved survival, although it appeared that the survival benefit with tamoxifen treatment was greatest for women.

7.3.9 Prevention of Hepatocellular Carcinoma in Cell Lines and Animal Models

It is beyond the purview of this review to discuss in detail chemoprevention of hepatocellular carcinoma in animal models or hepatocellular carcinoma cell lines. Nevertheless, there are multiple agents, which have shown activity against hepatocellular carcinoma raising hopes that these might be useful in humans in the future. An excellent review of phytochemicals in hepatocellular carcinoma chemoprevention in animal models is available (Mann et al. 2009) and is summarized in Table 7.1. Other agents, which have activity against hepatocellular carcinoma in animal models, are summarized in Table 7.2.

Table 7.1 Phytochemicals and other plant-derived agents in hepatocellular carcinoma (adapted from Mann et al. 2009)

Drug	Mechanism of action	Tested in	Results
Polyphenols			
Curcumin	Inhibits proliferation, and induces apoptosis in cell lines	Murine and rat models of chemical carcinogenesis	Decrease in preneoplastic foci, dysplastic nodules, and HCC
Resveratrol	Multiple	Chemical carcinogenesis model in rats	Reduced preneoplastic foci, reduced oxidative stress markers in liver
	Antioxidant, anti-inflammatory, antiproliferative, inhibits CYP450 and Phase II enzymes, apoptosis	Hepatoma cell lines transplanted into mice	
Epigallocatechin gallate (green tea polyphenols)	Inhibits growth and promotes apoptosis in cancer cell lines	Rat and mice models of chemical carcinogenesis	Decrease in preneoplastic foci, dysplastic nodules, and HCC
Caffeic acid	Reduces proliferation and viability of cell lines	Rat model of chemical carcinogenesis	Reduces preneoplastic foci
Ellagic acid	–	Rodent models of chemical and aflatoxin carcinogenesis	Reduces preneoplastic foci
Caffeine	Cell cycle arrest and apoptosis in cell lines	Rodent model of chemical carcinogenesis in rodents	Reduces preneoplastic foci
Capsaicin	Inhibits proliferation and induces apoptosis in cell lines	Rat model of chemical carcinogenesis	Reduces preneoplastic foci
Indol-3-carbinol	–	Rat models of chemical carcinogenesis	Reduces preneoplastic foci
Isothiocyanates	Inhibit proliferation and induce apoptosis in cell lines	Rat models of chemical carcinogenesis	Reduces preneoplastic foci
Oltipraz (synthetic derivative of dithiolthiones)	–	Rodent models of aflatoxin carcinogenesis	Reduces preneoplastic foci
Allium family (derived from garlic and onion)	Cell cycle arrest and apoptosis in cell lines	Rat models of chemical carcinogenesis	Reduces preneoplastic foci

(*continued*)

7

Table 7.1 (continued)

Drug	Mechanism of action	Tested in	Results
Monoterpenes			
Limonene	–	Rat models of chemical carcinogenesis	Reduces preneoplastic foci
Geraniol	–	Rat models of chemical carcinogenesis	Reduces preneoplastic foci
Flavonoids			
Quercetin	Inhibits activation of carcinogens; inhibits proliferation and induces apoptosis of cell lines	Rat models of chemical carcinogenesis	Reduces preneoplastic foci
Silymarin and silibinin	Inhibit growth and increase apoptosis in cell lines	Rat models of chemical carcinogenesis	Reduces preneoplastic foci
Genistein	Reduces proliferation and, angiogenesis; increases apoptosis	Epidemiology survey of HCC in humans	Epidemiology: reduced intake of genistein in patients who develop HCC
		Rat model of chemical carcinogenesis	Animal models: increases preneoplastic foci
Carotenoids			
Lutein	–	Rat models of chemical carcinogenesis	Reduces preneoplastic foci
Lycopene	Antioxidant; decreased proliferation and invasiveness of cell lines	Rat models of chemical carcinogenesis	Reduces preneoplastic foci

7.3.10 Phase II Trial of *S*-Adenosylmethionine in Hepatitis C Cirrhosis

S-adenosylmethionine (SAMe) is found in all cells in the body and is involved in the second most number of biochemical reactions after ATP. SAMe is a methyl donor for transmethylation reactions (donates methyl groups to DNA, RNA, and proteins), and is a precursor for phospholipids and for glutathione. Activity of the enzyme methionine adenosyl transferase (MAT), which synthesizes SAMe from methionine and ATP, is reduced in cirrhosis. Knockout of the *Mat1a* gene in mice reduces the amount of SAMe in the liver (the primary site of SAMe synthesis) and *Mat1a* knockout mice spontaneously develop hepatocellular carcinoma (Lu and Mato 2008). Furthermore, administration of SAMe to rats undergoing chemical carcinogenesis reduces the number of preneoplastic foci (Garcea et al. 1989). Similarly, intravenous administration of SAMe shortly after transplantation of H4IIE liver tumor cells into ACI rats reduced the development of hepatocellular carcinoma, although administration of SAMe after the HCC had already started growing in rats was ineffective in reducing tumor growth (Lu et al. 2009).

Based on these data, as well as extensive safety data on the use of SAMe in patients with liver disease, we began a Phase II clinical trial of SAMe in patients with hepatitis C cirrhosis. Patients without HCC at baseline were randomized to either placebo or to increasing doses of SAMe (up to 2.4 g/day) for a total treatment duration of 6 months. The primary outcome

Table 7.2 Other chemical agents that prevent hepatocarcinogenesis in cell culture and/or animal models

	Mechanism of action	Tested in	Results	Reference
Bicyclol	–	Humans with hepatitis B or C (China)	Inhibit hepatitis B and C virus; improve liver function and histology	Liu et al. (2006)
	–	Rats with DEN carcinogenesis	Reduced number of premalignant foci, and markers of neoplasia (GST-P, AFP, N-ras, c-myc)	Zhu et al. (2006)
Amiloride	Inhibition of cell proliferation	Chemical carcinogenesis in rats	Reduced preneoplastic foci	Tatsuta et al. (1997)
Wnt-1 signaling blockade (anti-Wnt-1 antibody)	Decreased proliferation and apoptosis of cell lines	HuH7 xenograft model	Intratumoral injection of anti-WNT-1 antibody reduced tumor growth	Wei et al. (2009)
Butyric acid (histone deacetylase inhibitor)	Alters gene expression	Chemical carcinogenesis in rats	Reduced preneoplastic foci	Kuroiwa-Trzmielina et al. (2009)
COX-2 inhibitors (e.g., Celocoxib)	COX-2 mediated: Apoptosis, antiproliferative, inhibits	DEN rats	Reduces preneoplastic foci	Reviewed in Wu (2006)
	ERK1/2,COX-2 independent: PPAR-gamma, PPAR-alpha, EGFR signaling	Xenographs into SCID mice	Reduces HCC growth SCID mice	
S-adenosylmethionine (SAMe)	Increases SAMe content in liver Inhibits mitogenic effects of growth factors; regulates apoptosis in liver cancer cells	*Mat1a* knockout mice, rodent chemical carcinogenesis	HCC develops in *Mat1a* knockout mouse SAMe administration reduces preneoplastic foci in DEN hepatocellular carcinogenesis model; reduced HCC growth if administered soon after transplant of H4IIE tumor cells into rats	Lu and Mato (2008)

(*continued*)

Table 7.2 (continued)

	Mechanism of action	Tested in	Results	Reference
Aurora kinase inhibitor (PHA-739358)	Inhibits proliferation of cell lines	HCC xenographs	Inhibited growth of xenographs	Benten et al. (2009)
Selenium	Increased antioxidants; inhibition of proliferation and increased apoptosis in cell lines	Human and animal carcinogenesis studies	Humans: reduces HCC in humans with hepatitis B cirrhosis Animal models: reduces size of preneoplastic foci	Reviewed in Rayman (2005)
Spirulina platensis (a cyanobacterium)	Inhibition of proliferation and increased apoptosis in cell lines	Rat models of chemical carcinogenesis	Reduces preneoplastic foci	Ismail et al. (2009)
Omega-3 fatty acids (fish oils)	–	Rat models of chemical carcinogenesis	Reduces preneoplastic foci	Rahman et al. (1999). Kim et al. (2000)
Pioglitazone (PPAR-gamma agonist	–	Rat models of chemical carcinogenesis	Reduces preneoplastic foci	Borbath et al. (2007)
Rifampicin	Inhibits angiogenesis	Human (six patients), animal model and cell culture	One of six patients developed HCC Reduced growth of xenographs Inhibits proliferation of endothelial cells	Shichiri et al. (2009)
miRNA (miR-26a)	Cell cycle arrest	Transgenic mouse model of HCC	Adenoviral mediated delivery of miR-26a prevented growth of HCC in animal model	Kota et al. (2009)

variable was change in serum level of alpha fetoprotein. At this time, approximately 50 patients have been enrolled, with a goal of 100.

7.4 Conclusions

Hepatitis C is a common cause of hepatocellular carcinoma throughout the world. Because of the increase in hepatitis C infections during the 1970s and 1980s in the United States, there has been an increase in the incidence of hepatocellular carcinoma during the past 3 decades, with an expectation of continued increase in the next few years. Hepatocellular carcinoma is frequent in other countries, possibly related of spread of HCV by iatrogenic means in the past.

Curing hepatitis C infection in patients with cirrhosis reduces the risk of developing hepatocellular carcinoma. Several noncurative treatments have prevented the development of hepatocellular carcinoma in prospective human trials in patients with cirrhosis (predominantly from hepatitis C). The drugs used in these trials have been safe and presumably relatively inexpensive. Several uncontrolled trials have demonstrated a marked reduction in the incidence of hepatocellular carcinoma. In addition, relatively safe drugs have reduced the occurrence of secondary hepatocellular carcinoma and/or prolonged life in patients with hepatocellular carcinoma. Overall, these studies raise the possibility that safe and relatively inexpensive drugs are available for use in prospective, placebo-controlled chemoprevention of hepatocellular carcinoma trials in patients with chronic hepatitis C.

Multiple drugs, both synthetic and naturally occurring, have antitumor effects in animal models of carcinogenesis. Many of these drugs appear to be safe and are potential candidates for future chemoprevention studies in hepatitis C cirrhosis. Finally, results are awaited on the Phase II study of SAMe treatment in patients with hepatitis C cirrhosis, which is currently in progress.

References

Altekruse SF, McGlynn KA et al (2009) Hepatocellular carcinoma incidence, mortality, and survival trends in the United States from 1975 to 2005. J Clin Oncol 27(9):1485–1491

Arase Y, Ikeda K et al (1997) The long term efficacy of glycyrrhizin in chronic hepatitis C patients. Cancer 79(8):1494–1500

Backus LI, Boothroyd DB et al (2007) Predictors of response of US veterans to treatment for the hepatitis C virus. Hepatology 46(1):37–47

Benten D, Keller G et al (2009) Aurora kinase inhibitor PHA-739358 suppresses growth of hepatocellular carcinoma in vitro and in a xenograft mouse model. Neoplasia 11(9):934–944

Bjelakovic G, Nikolova D et al (2004) Antioxidant supplements for prevention of gastrointestinal cancers: a systematic review and meta-analysis. Lancet 364(9441):1219–1228

Blonski W, Reddy KR (2008) Hepatitis C virus infection and hepatocellular carcinoma. Clin Liver Dis 12(3):661–674, x

Borbath I, Leclercq I et al (2007) The PPARgamma agonist pioglitazone inhibits early neoplastic occurrence in the rat liver. Eur J Cancer 43(11): 1755–1763

Bosch FX, Ribes J et al (2005) Epidemiology of hepatocellular carcinoma. Clin Liver Dis 9(2):191–211, v

Bravi F, Bosetti C et al (2007) Coffee drinking and hepatocellular carcinoma risk: a meta-analysis. Hepatology 46(2):430–435

Bravi F, Bosetti C et al (2009) Coffee drinking and hepatocellular carcinoma: an update. Hepatology 50(4):1317–1318

Bruix J, Sherman M (2005) Management of hepatocellular carcinoma. Hepatology 42(5):1208–1236

Bruno S, Stroffolini T et al (2007) Sustained virological response to interferon alpha is associated with improved outcome in HCV-related cirrhosis: a retrospective study. Hepatology 45(3):579–587

Choo QL, Kuo G et al (1989) Isolation of a cDNA clone derived from a blood-borne non-A, non-B viral hepatitis genome. Science 244(4902):359–362

7

Davis GL, Balart LA et al (1989) Treatment of chronic hepatitis C with recombinant interferon alfa. A multicenter randomized, controlled trial. Hepatitis Interventional Therapy Group. N Engl J Med 321(22):1501–1506

Davis GL, Alter MJ et al (2010) Aging of hepatitis C virus (HCV)-infected persons in the United States: a multiple cohort model of HCV prevalence and disease progression. Gastroenterology 138(2):513–521, 521 e511–516

Di Bisceglie AM, Osmack P et al (2005) Chemoprevention of hepatocellular carcinoma: use of tamoxifen in an animal model of hepatocarcinogenesis. J Lab Clin Med 145(3):134–138

Di Bisceglie AM, Shiffman ML et al (2008) Prolonged therapy of advanced chronic hepatitis C with low-dose peginterferon. N Engl J Med 359(23):2429–2441

Dimitroulopoulos D, Xinopoulos D et al (2007) Long acting octreotide in the treatment of advanced hepatocellular cancer and overexpression of somatostatin receptors: randomized placebo-controlled trial. World J Gastroenterol 13(23): 3164–3170

El-Serag HB, Rudolph KL (2007) Hepatocellular carcinoma: epidemiology and molecular carcinogenesis. Gastroenterology 132(7):2557–2576

Feinstone SM, Kapikian AZ et al (1975) Transfusion-associated hepatitis not due to viral hepatitis type A or B. N Engl J Med 292(15):767–770

Freedman ND, Everhart JE et al (2009) Coffee intake is associated with lower rates of liver disease progression in chronic hepatitis C. Hepatology 50(5): 1360–1369

Garcea R, Daino L et al (1989) Inhibition of promotion and persistent nodule growth by S-adenosyl-L-methionine in rat liver carcinogenesis: role of remodeling and apoptosis. Cancer Res 49(7): 1850–1856

George SL, Bacon BR et al (2009) Clinical, virologic, histologic, and biochemical outcomes after successful HCV therapy: a 5-year follow-up of 150 patients. Hepatology 49(3):729–738

Habu D, Shiomi S et al (2004) Role of vitamin K2 in the development of hepatocellular carcinoma in women with viral cirrhosis of the liver. JAMA 292(3):358–361

Hirayama C, Okumura M et al (1989) A multicenter randomized controlled clinical trial of Shosaiko-to in chronic active hepatitis. Gastroenterol Jpn 24(6):715–719

Ismail MF, Ali DA et al (2009) Chemoprevention of rat liver toxicity and carcinogenesis by Spirulina. Int J Biol Sci 5(4):377–387

Kim Y, Ji SK et al (2000) Modulation of liver microsomal monooxygenase system by dietary n-6/n-3 ratios in rat hepatocarcinogenesis. Nutr Cancer 37(1):65–72

Kojima S, Okuno M et al (2004) Acyclic retinoid in the chemoprevention of hepatocellular carcinoma (review). Int J Oncol 24(4):797–805

Kota J, Chivukula RR et al (2009) Therapeutic microRNA delivery suppresses tumorigenesis in a murine liver cancer model. Cell 137(6):1005–1017

Kouroumalis E, Skordilis P et al (1998) Treatment of hepatocellular carcinoma with octreotide: a randomised controlled study. Gut 42(3):442–447

Kuo G, Choo QL et al (1989) An assay for circulating antibodies to a major etiologic virus of human non-A, non-B hepatitis. Science 244(4902):362–364

Kuroiwa-Trzmielina J, de Conti A et al (2009) Chemoprevention of rat hepatocarcinogenesis with histone deacetylase inhibitors: efficacy of tributyrin, a butyric acid prodrug. Int J Cancer 124(11):2520–2527

La Vecchia C (2005) Coffee, liver enzymes, cirrhosis and liver cancer. J Hepatol 42(4):444–446

Larsson SC, Wolk A (2007) Coffee consumption and risk of liver cancer: a meta-analysis. Gastroenterology 132(5):1740–1745

Liu Q, Song Y et al (2006) A useful agent for chemoprevention of hepatocellular carcinoma? Cancer Biol Ther 5(12):1674–1676

Llovet JM, Ricci S et al (2008) Sorafenib in advanced hepatocellular carcinoma. N Engl J Med 359(4):378–390

Lok AS, Seeff LB et al (2009) Incidence of hepatocellular carcinoma and associated risk factors in hepatitis C-related advanced liver disease. Gastroenterology 136(1):138–148

Lu SC, Mato JM (2008) S-Adenosylmethionine in cell growth, apoptosis and liver cancer. J Gastroenterol Hepatol 23(Suppl 1):S73–77

Lu SC, Ramani K et al (2009) S-adenosylmethionine in the chemoprevention and treatment of hepatocellular carcinoma in a rat model. Hepatology 50(2):462–471

Manesis EK, Giannoulis G et al (1995) Treatment of hepatocellular carcinoma with combined suppression and inhibition of sex hormones: a randomized, controlled trial. Hepatology 21(6): 1535–1542

Mann CD, Neal CP et al (2009) Phytochemicals as potential chemopreventive and chemotherapeutic agents in hepatocarcinogenesis. Eur J Cancer Prev 18(1):13–25

Modi AA, Feld JJ et al (2010) Increased caffeine consumption is associated with reduced hepatic fibrosis. Hepatology 51(1):201–209

Moriwaki H, Shimizu M et al (2007) Chemoprevention of liver carcinogenesis with retinoids: basic and clinical aspects. Hepatol Res 37(Suppl 2): S299–302

Muto Y, Moriwaki H et al (1996) Prevention of second primary tumors by an acyclic retinoid, polyprenoic acid, in patients with hepatocellular carcinoma. Hepatoma Prevention Study Group. N Engl J Med 334(24):1561–1567

Muto Y, Moriwaki H et al (1999) Prevention of second primary tumors by an acyclic retinoid in patients with hepatocellular carcinoma. N Engl J Med 340(13):1046–1047

Nishino H (2007) Prevention of hepatocellular carcinoma in chronic viral hepatitis patients with cirrhosis by carotenoid mixture. Recent Results Cancer Res 174:67–71

Nishino H (2009) Phytochemicals in hepatocellular cancer prevention. Nutr Cancer 61(6):789–791

Nishino H, Murakoshi M et al (2009) Cancer prevention by carotenoids. Arch Biochem Biophys 483(2):165–168

Oka H, Yamamoto S et al (1995) Prospective study of chemoprevention of hepatocellular carcinoma with Sho-saiko-to (TJ-9). Cancer 76(5):743–749

Parkin DM (2001) Global cancer statistics in the year 2000. Lancet Oncol 2(9):533–543

Rahman KM, Sugie S et al (1999) Modulating effects of diets high in omega-3 and omega-6 fatty acids in initiation and postinitiation stages of diethylnitrosamine-induced hepatocarcinogenesis in rats. Jpn J Cancer Res 90(1):31–39

Rayman MP (2005) Selenium in cancer prevention: a review of the evidence and mechanism of action. Proc Nutr Soc 64(4):527–542

Ruhl CE, Everhart JE (2005a) Coffee and caffeine consumption reduce the risk of elevated serum alanine aminotransferase activity in the United States. Gastroenterology 128(1):24–32

Ruhl CE, Everhart JE (2005b) Coffee and tea consumption are associated with a lower incidence of chronic liver disease in the United States. Gastroenterology 129(6):1928–1936

Seeff LB (2009) The history of the "natural history" of hepatitis C (1968–2009). Liver Int 29(Suppl 1):89–99

Shichiri M, Fukai N et al (2009) Rifampicin as an oral angiogenesis inhibitor targeting hepatic cancers. Cancer Res 69(11):4760–4768

Shiffman ML, Morishima C et al (2009) Effect of HCV RNA suppression during peginterferon alfa-2a maintenance therapy on clinical outcomes in the Halt-C trial. Gastroenterology 50(Suppl 1):S22

Shimizu M, Takai K et al (2009) Strategy and mechanism for the prevention of hepatocellular carcinoma: phosphorylated retinoid X receptor alpha is a critical target for hepatocellular carcinoma chemoprevention. Cancer Sci 100(3):369–374

Takami A, Nakao S et al (1999) Successful therapy of myelodysplastic syndrome with menatetrenone, a vitamin K2 analog. Int J Hematol 69(1):24–26

Tamori A, Habu D et al (2007) Potential role of vitamin K(2) as a chemopreventive agent against hepatocellular carcinoma. Hepatol Res 37(Suppl 2):S303–307

Tanaka T, Nishikawa A et al (1990) Inhibitory effects of chlorogenic acid, reserpine, polyprenoic acid (E-5166), or coffee on hepatocarcinogenesis in rats and hamsters. Basic Life Sci 52:429–440

Tarao K, Fujiyama S et al (2005) Ursodiol use is possibly associated with lower incidence of hepatocellular carcinoma in hepatitis C virus-associated liver cirrhosis. Cancer Epidemiol Biomark Prev 14(1):164–169

Tatsuta M, Iishi H et al (1997) Chemoprevention by amiloride against experimental hepatocarcinogenesis induced by N-nitrosomorpholine in Sprague-Dawley rats. Cancer Lett 119(1): 109–113

Veldt BJ, Heathcote EJ et al (2007) Sustained virologic response and clinical outcomes in patients with chronic hepatitis C and advanced fibrosis. Ann Intern Med 147(10):677–684

Wei W, Chua MS et al (2009) Blockade of Wnt-1 signaling leads to anti-tumor effects in hepatocellular carcinoma cells. Mol Cancer 8:76

Wu T (2006) Cyclooxygenase-2 in hepatocellular carcinoma. Cancer Treat Rev 32(1):28–44

Zhu B, Liu GT et al (2006) Chemoprevention of bicyclol against hepatic preneoplastic lesions. Cancer Biol Ther 5(12):1665–1673

Nutritional Aspects of Primary Prostate Cancer Prevention

8

Hans-Peter Schmid, Claus Fischer, Daniel S. Engeler, Marcelo L. Bendhack, and Bernd J. Schmitz-Dräger

Abstract There are three well-known and indisputable risk factors for development of prostate cancer, namely heredity, ethnic origin, and increasing age. Geographic variations in incidence rates are considerable and, therefore, it has been suggested that environmental factors may also play a role. Data from migration studies clearly show that men with the same genetic background raised in different environments present the risk of the disease associated with their country of residency. Prostate cancer is a good candidate for studies on primary prevention due to several specific features such as high prevalence, long latency, hormonal dependency, serum markers for monitoring (prostate specific antigen), and histological precursor lesions (prostatic intraepithelial neoplasia). Nutritional factors that may influence the disease include total energy intake (as reflected by body mass index), dietary fat, cooked meat, micronutrients and vitamins (carotenoids, retinoids, vitamins C, D and E), fruit and vegetable intake, minerals (calcium, selenium), and phytoestrogens (isoflavonoids, flavonoids, lignans). Most studies reported to date are case–control analysis. The selenium and vitamin E cancer prevention trial (SELECT), however, is a population-based, prospective, randomized clinical trial to examine the effect of selenium and vitamin E alone or in combination on prostate cancer risk reduction. The trial was discontinued recently as there was no evidence of a benefit from either agent. Nevertheless, lifestyle changes could be recommended to men at risk for developing clinical prostate cancer.

H.-P. Schmid (✉) and D.S. Engeler
Department of Urology, Kantonsspital, 9007 St. Gallen, Switzerland
e-mail: hans-peter.schmid@kssg.ch

C. Fischer
Department of Urology, Krankenhaus Hohe Warte, 95445 Bayreuth, Germany

M.L. Bendhack
PUC Catholic, University of Parana Nossa Sra. das Graca Hospital, 80030-200, Curitiba, Brazil

B.J. Schmitz-Dräger
Euromed Clinic, Europa-Allee 1, 90763 Fürth, Germany

8.1 Introduction

There are three well-known and indisputable risk factors for prostate cancer, namely increasing age, ethnic origin, and hereditary/familial factors (Heidenreich et al. 2008). International variations in incidence rates for the disease are

H.-J. Senn and F. Otto (eds.), *Clinical Cancer Prevention*, Recent Results in Cancer Research 188, DOI: 10.1007/978-3-642-10858-7_8, considerable and it has been suggested that environmental factors may also play a major role. Indeed, data from migration studies clearly demonstrate that the incidence for Asian men increases significantly when moving from their country of origin to the United States.

Prostatic adenocarcinoma is an ideal candidate for prevention because of several important features including high prevalence of the disease. Endocrine and hormonal dependency makes it susceptible to pharmacological manipulations. Progression is very slow with a long latency period (Schmid et al. 1993). Histological precursor lesions such as prostatic intraepithelial neoplasia (PIN) take about 10 years to develop into early invasive tumor, with clinically significant cancer occurring some 3–4 years later. Prostate-specific antigen (PSA) is a good serum marker for clinical monitoring of the disease.

There are, on the other hand, multiple factors potentially influencing the results of trials and making analysis of data more difficult. Among them are validity of studies (case–control, cohort, interventional) (Table 8.1), the follow-up interval in the interventional and most cohort studies, validity of questionnaires, hereditary factors, data from different ethnic backgrounds, correlation between nutrition and lifestyle, and interaction between several nutritional compounds (Schmitz-Dräger et al. 2001).

Table 8.1 Data on dietary and nutritional factors according to evidence levels

Level Ia	No data
Level Ib	Selenium, vitamin E, vitamin C
Level IIa	Lycopene
Level IIb	Dietary fat, vitamin E, rye, soya, and phytoestrogens
Level III	Saturated fat, beta-carotene
Cochrane collaboration	

8.2 Dietary/Nutritional Factors

8.2.1 Dietary Fat

High calorie intake has often been associated with an increased risk of prostate cancer. However, the interaction between various compounds (total fat, animal fat, saturated or unsaturated fatty acids, cholesterol, triglycerides, omega-3 fatty acids) is very complex (Wuermli et al. 2005). Theoretically, high energy intake may stimulate the sympathetic nervous system and basal metabolism and consecutively increase IGF-1 release, thus leading to increased mitosis and cell proliferation (Meyer et al. 1999). The majority of case–control and cohort studies report a positive association between fat consumption and prostate cancer with a relative risk around 2.

8.2.2 Obesity

Contradictory findings on the role of obesity in the development of prostate carcinoma have been obtained from different studies with problematic methodology (Lucia et al. 2007). Although numerous studies have reported on a relationship between obesity and the occurrence of more aggressive or more advanced prostate carcinoma – at least in patients aged between 65 and 75 years – it is now assumed that the greater plasma volume in overweight men leads to a higher dilution of PSA and therefore to a lower concentration, thus delaying diagnosis.

8.2.3 Micronutrients

Carotenoids are a group of complex unsaturated hydrocarbons occurring as pigment in plants such as carrots (alpha-, beta-, gamma-carotene) and tomatoes (lycopene). Some carotenoids, but not lycopene, are precursors of vitamin A and they have been shown to act as antioxidants and inhibitors of IGF-1. Giovannucci (1999) reviewed 72 studies concerning intake of tomatoes and tomato-based products and blood lycopene levels in relation to the risk of various cancers. An inverse association was identified in 57 reports and 35 of them were statistically significant. The evidence for a benefit was strongest for tumors of the prostate, lung, and stomach. Conversely, no study indicated that intake of tomatoes or a high serum lycopene level led to an increased risk of cancer of any site.

8.2.4 Vitamins

Numerous studies could demonstrate an inverse correlation between intake of vitamins and incidence of various types of malignant tumors. Of special interest with regard to prostate cancer were vitamins A, C, D, and E.

Vitamin A (retinol) and its precursor (betacarotene) are found in foods of animal origin (liver, fish oil) and in carrots and green vegetables (spinach, broccoli), respectively. They act as antioxidants by suppressing the carcinogenic potential of free radicals, enhance the immune system, and induce cellular differentiation. Dose-related side effects include hepatotoxicity, central nervous system changes, and mucocutaneous dryness and, therefore, hamper their use in clinical trials (Heinonen et al. 1998).

Vitamin C is a water-soluble antioxidant in fruits and vegetables. The majority of case–control and cohort studies failed to demonstrate any correlation between vitamin C intake or plasma concentrations and occurrence of prostate cancer. The Physicians' Health Study II randomized controlled trial also did not show an effect of vitamin C on total cancer or prostate cancer compared with placebo (Gaziano et al. 2009).

Calcitriol (1,25 dihydroxyvitamin D3) is the active form of vitamin D and is responsible for calcium metabolism in kidneys, bone, and gut. A favorable impact of ultraviolet radiation (sun exposure), which is the main source of vitamin D, on the incidence of prostate cancer has been postulated (Hanchette and Schwartz 1992). In primary cultures of prostatic tissues derived from prostate cancer patients, vitamin D3 carried out antiproliferative effects (Peehl et al. 1994). However, the role of vitamin D in prostate cancer promotion and prevention is still controversial.

Vitamin E (alpha-tocopherol) is a fat-soluble potent intracellular antioxidant occurring in lettuce, watercress, and cotton- and hemp-seed oil. In the Finnish alpha-tocopherol beta-carotene (ATBC) trial, 29,133 male smokers aged 50–69 years were randomly assigned to receive alpha-tocopherol (50 mg), beta-carotene (20 mg), both agents, or placebo daily for 5–8 years (Heinonen et al. 1998). However, in this study prostate cancer was only looked at as a secondary end point. A 32% decrease in the incidence and a 41% decrease in mortality from prostate cancer were observed among the subjects receiving alpha-tocopherol compared with those not receiving it. Notably, among men receiving beta-carotene, prostate cancer incidence was 23% higher and mortality was 15% higher compared with those not receiving it. Contrary to the Finnish study, the Physicians' Health Study II from the United States found no impact of vitamin E on the incidence of total or prostate cancer (Gaziano et al. 2009).

8.2.5 Minerals

Conversion of vitamin D to the active form 1,25 dihydroxyvitamin D3 is suppressed by high consumption of dietary calcium (milk, cheese). Furthermore, low serum calcium levels stimulate the secretion of parathyroid hormone which promotes the conversion of vitamin D to calcitriol. From a clinical point of view, calcium has been found in excess levels to be associated with an increased rate of prostate cancer progression.

8

Selenium, a trace element occurring predominantly as selenomethionine in dietary supplements (bread, cereals, fish, chicken, meat), is a key component of a number of functional selenoproteins required for normal health. In a double-blind cancer prevention trial, 974 men with a history of basal cell or squamous cell carcinoma were randomized to either receive 200 µg selenium daily or placebo for a mean of 4.5 years (Clark et al. 1998). Selenium treatment was associated with a 63% reduction in the secondary endpoint of prostate cancer incidence, but the number of cases was rather low. Long-term selenium intake can be determined in toenails. In a nested case–control study within the Health Professionals Follow-Up Study, high levels of selenium in toenails were correlated with a reduced risk for advanced prostate cancer (Yoshizawa et al. 1998). A more recent prospective case–control study did not find a statistically significant difference in toenail selenium levels of patients with newly diagnosed prostate cancer and matched controls (Lipsky et al. 2004). The National Cancer Institute launched a large randomized trial (SELECT study) with four arms to compare selenium (200 µg) plus vitamin E (400 IU) to either agent alone or to placebo. Included were 35,533 men from 427 sites in the United States, Canada, and Puerto Rico with a PSA level of 4 ng/mL or less and an unsuspicious digital rectal examination. As of October 2008, median overall follow-up was 5.5 years. Hazard ratios for prostate cancer were 1.13 for vitamin E, 1.04 for selenium, and 1.05 for selenium+vitamin E versus placebo (Lippman et al. 2009). There were no significant differences in any other prespecified cancer end points. There were statistically nonsignificant increased risks of prostate cancer in the vitamin E group and type 2 diabetes mellitus in the selenium group but not in the selenium + vitamin E group.

8.2.6 Phytoestrogens

The major categories of phytoestrogens include isoflavonoids (genistein, daidzein), flavonoids (quercetin), and lignans (enterolactone). The first two groups are found in vegetables such as beans, peas, and especially soy and in fruits; lignans also occur in grains, cereals, and linseeds. The putative biological effects of phytoestrogens are listed in Table 8.2. In geographic areas with low prostate cancer incidence (Asia, southern Europe) diets are rich in phytoestrogens, which has been confirmed by higher serum levels or urinary concentrations of phytoestrogens compared to Western countries (Adlercreutz et al. 1993). The favorable antitumoral effects of various soy-derived products have been demonstrated in experimental studies; however, clinical data are sparse and assessment of dietary phytoestrogen intake is complex. In an analysis of data from 59 countries, prostate cancer mortality was related to food consumption, tobacco use, socioeconomic factors, reproductive factors, and health indicators (Hebert et al. 1998). Mortality rates were inversely associated with estimated intake of cereals, nuts, oilseed and fish, and soy products were found to be significantly protective.

Table 8.2 Potential mechanisms of phytoestrogens on prostatic epithelial cells

Increase of SHBG serum concentration and subsequent decrease of free testosterone through binding to liver estrogen receptors
Decrease of DNA synthesis through inhibition of tyrosine kinase an topoisomerase
Decrease of the effects of free radicals through antioxidant properties
Inhibition of cytochrome P450 activation
Neoangiogenesis inhibition
Inhibition of intraprostatic testosterone metabolism through inhibition of 5-alpha-reductase and aromatase

SHBG Sex hormone binding globulin
Adapted from Schmitz-Dräger et al. 2001

8.2.7 Diabetes Mellitus

The presence of diabetes mellitus obviously does not increase the risk of developing prostate carcinoma, unlike other tumor disorders. On the contrary, meta-analyses show that diabetes sufferers have a lower risk of developing prostate carcinoma (Kasper and Giovannucci 2006).

8.3 American Cancer Society (ACS) Guideline

The four principal recommendations of the American guidelines are (Kushi et al. 2006):

A. Try to maintain a healthy weight.
B. Take regular physical exercise.
C. Maintain a healthy diet with a focus on fruit and vegetables.
D. Reduce alcohol intake.

8.3.1 A: Try to Maintain a Healthy Weight

- Try to maintain a healthy balance between calorie intake and physical activity.
- Avoid or reduce overweight and try to maintain your ideal weight once you have reached it.
- The healthiest way to reduce the calorie intake is to reduce the intake of sugar, saturated and trans fats, and alcohol, or to refrain from them altogether.

All these foods are of high calorie or have too few or no essential nutritional elements such as vitamins, minerals, or fiber. Examples of unfavorable foods that should be avoided are deep-fried and fried dishes, biscuits, cakes, sugar products, ice creams, and soft drinks.

8.3.2 B: Take Regular Physical Exercise

At least 30 min of moderate to intense physical exercise in addition to the usual daily activities on at least 5 days each week are recommended. 45–60 min is the ideal target. Moderate exercise is understood to be the degree of exertion achieved by fast walking, such as dancing, slow cycling, playing golf, mowing the lawn, or gardening. Intense physical activity involves the use of larger muscle groups, increases the pulse and breathing, and causes sweating, e.g. jogging or running, aerobics, swimming, fast cycling, or heavy garden work. Increasing everyday activities such as climbing stairs instead of using a lift, or walking or cycling instead of driving, is equivalent to doing sporting activities.

8.3.3 C: Maintain a Healthy Diet with a Focus on Fruit and Vegetables

- Eat different fruits and vegetables every day.
- Eat whole wheat rather than refined wheat products.
- Eat only small quantities of meat products and red meat.

A large cohort study showed a relationship between the development of prostate carcinoma and the intake of barbecued or heavily browned meat products in particular.

8.3.4 D: Reduce Alcohol Intake

Men should not have more than two alcoholic drinks per day. One "drink" (12 g alcohol) corresponds to 330 mL 5% proof beer, 40 mL 40% proof spirits, 140 mL 12% proof wine or sparkling wine, or 70 mL 20% proof fortified wine/aperitif/liqueur.

Several studies have, however, agreed in showing that alcohol intake appears to have a marginal effect at the most on the development of prostate carcinoma. What must nevertheless be borne in mind is that alcohol is high in calories and that a high intake has an effect on body weight.

8

8.4 Conclusions

There are currently no conclusive study outcomes with respect to nutritional prevention of prostate cancer that meet the criteria of evidence-based medicine. Despite this lack of results from prospective trials, lifestyle changes can be recommended to men at risk for developing clinical prostate cancer (Heidenreich et al. 2008). These measures may include balanced food intake (Mediterranean style) and physical activity (Schmitz-Dräger et al. 2009).

References

Adlercreutz H, Markkanen H, Watanabe S (1993) Plasma concentrations of phyto-oestrogens in Japanese men. Lancet 342:1209–1210

Clark LC, Dalkin B, Krongrad A, Combs GF Jr, Turnbull BW, Slate EH, Witherington R, Herlong JH, Janosko E, Carpenter D, Borosso C, Falk S, Rounder J (1998) Decreased incidence of prostate cancer with selenium supplementation: results of a double-blind cancer prevention trial. Br J Urol 81:730–734

Gaziano JM, Glynn RJ, Christen WG, Kurth T, Belanger C, MacFadyen J, Bubes V, Manson JE, Sesso HD, Buring JE (2009) Vitamins E and C in the prevention of prostate and toal cancer in men: the physicians' health study II randomized controlled trial. JAMA 301:52–62

Giovannucci E (1999) Tomatoes, tomato-based products, lycopene, and cancer: review of the epidemiologic literature. J Natl Cancer Inst 91:317–331

Hanchette CL, Schwartz GG (1992) Geographic patterns of prostate cancer mortality. Evidence for a protective effect of ultraviolet radiation Cancer 70:2861–2869

Hebert JR, Hurley TG, Olendzki BC, Teas J, Ma Y, Hampl JS (1998) Nutritional and socioeconomic factors in relation to prostate cancer mortality: a cross-national study. J Natl Cancer Inst 90: 1637–1647

Heidenreich A, Aus G, Bolla M, Joniau S, Matveev VB, Schmid H-P, Zattoni F (2008) EAU guidelines on prostate cancer. Eur Urol 53:68–80

Heinonen OP, Albanes D, Virtamo J, Taylor PR, Huttunen JK, Hartman AM, Haapakoski J, Malila N, Rautalahti M, Ripatti S, Maenpaa H, Teerenhovi L, Koss L, Virolainen M, Edwards BK (1998) Prostate cancer and supplementation with alpha-tocopherol and beta-carotene: incidence and mortality in a controlled trial. J Natl Cancer Inst 90:440–446

Kasper JS, Giovannucci E (2006) A meta-analysis of diabetes mellitus and the risk of prostate cancer. Cancer Epidemiol Biomarkers Prev 15:2056–2062

Kushi LH, Byers T, Doyle C, Bandera EV, McCullough M, McTiernan A, Gansler T, Andrews KS (2006) Thun MJ; American Cancer Society 2006 Nutrition and Physical Activity Guidelines Advisory Committee. CA Cancer J Clin 56:254–281

Lippman SM, Klein EA, Goodman PJ, Lucia MS, Thompson IM, Ford LG, Parnes HL, Minasian LM, Gaziano JM, Hartline JA, Parsons JK, Bearden JD 3rd, Crawford ED, Goodman GE, Claudio J, Winquist E, Cook ED, Karp DD, Walther P, Lieber MM, Kristal AR, Darke AK, Arnold KB, Ganz PA, Santella RM, Albanes D, Taylor PR, Probstfield JL, Jagpal TJ, Crowley JJ, Meyskens FL Jr, Baker LH, Coltman CA Jr (2009) Effect of selenium and vitamin E on risk of prostate cancer and other cancers: the Selenium and Vitamin E Cancer Prevention Trial (SELECT). JAMA 302:39–51

Lipsky K, Zigeuner R, Zischka M, Schips L, Pummer K, Rehak P, Hubmer G (2004) Selenium levels of patients with newly diagnosed prostate cancer compared with control group. Urology 62:912–916

Lucia MS, Epstein JI, Goodman PJ, Darke AK, Reuter VE, Civantos F, Tangen CM, Parnes HL, Lippman SM, La Rosa FG, Kattan MW, Crawford ED, Fort LG, Coltman CA Jr, Thompson IM (2007) Finasteride and high-grade prostate cancer in the Prostate Cancer Prevention Trial. J Natl Cancer Inst 99:1375–1383

Meyer F, Bairati I, Shadmani R, Fradet Y, Moore L (1999) Dietary fat and prostate cancer survival. Cancer Causes Control 10:245–251

Peehl DM, Skowronski RJ, Leung GK, Wong ST, Stamey TA, Feldman D (1994) Antiproliferative effects of 1, 25 dihydroxyvitamin D3 on primary cultures of human prostatic cells. Cancer Res 54:805–810

Schmid H-P, McNeal JE, Stamey TA (1993) Clinical observations on the doubling time of prostate cancer. Eur Urol 23(suppl 2):60–63

Schmitz-Dräger BJ, Eichholzer M, Beiche B, Ebert T (2001) Nutrition and prostate cancer. Urol Int 67:1–11

Schmitz-Dräger B, Fiebrandt H-J, Lümmen G. Prävention und Ernährung. In: Wirth M, Weißbach L, Ackermann R, Alberti W, Albrecht C, Göckel-Beining B, Fröhner M, Hinkelbein W, Miller K, Rübben H, Wiegel T, Wolff J, Wörmann B (Hrsg.): Interdisziplinäre Leitlinie der Qualität S3 zur Früherkennung, Diagnose und Therapie der verschiedenen Stadien des Prostatakarzinoms. DGU, Düsseldorf, 2009, S. 19–22

Wuermli L, Joerger M, Henz S, Schmid H-P, Riesen WF, Thomas G, Krek W, Cerny T, Gillessen S (2005) Hypertriglyceridemia as a possible risk factor for prostate cancer. Prostate Cancer Prostatic Dis 8:316–320

Yoshizawa K, Willett WC, Morris SJ, Stampfer MJ, Spiegelman D, Rimm EB, Giovannucci E (1998) Study of prediagnostic selenium level in toenails and the risk of advanced prostate cancer. J Natl Cancer Inst 90:1219–1224

Prostate Cancer Prevention with 5 Alpha-Reductase Inhibitors

9

Dipen J. Parekh

Testosterone gets converted into the more potent 5-[alpha]-dihydrotestosterone by 5-[alpha]-reductase. dihydrotestosterone (DHT) controls prostate mitotic activity and potentially prostate carcinogenesis. Interventions that inhibit 5-[alpha]-reductase have potential as preventive agents for prostate cancer. Two 5-[alpha]-reductase inhibitors (5ARI), finasteride, and dutasteride, are currently available for commercial use. Finasteride is selective for the type 2 isoenzyme, which reduces the level of dihydrotestosterone (DHT) by 65–70% (McConnell et al. 1992). Dutasteride inhibits both type 1 and type 2 isoenzymes and reduces the level of DHT by approximately 90% (Clark et al. 2004). So far only one randomized trial of 5ARIs as chemopreventive agents has assessed the effect of finasteride on the prevalence of biopsy-proven prostate cancer – the Prostate Cancer Prevention trial (PCPT) (Thompson et al. 2003). Results from another placebo-controlled phase III clinical trial with dutasteride – the Reduction by Dutasteride of Prostate Cancer Events trial (REDUCE trial) are expected to be published in the near future (Andriole et al. 2004).

D.J. Parekh
Robotic Surgery, Department of Urology,
University of Texas Health Sciences Center
at San Antonio, San Antonio, TX, USA
e-mail: parekhd@uthscsa.edu

9.1 Rationale for the Chemoprevention of Prostate Cancer

Prostate cancer is a leading cause of cancer and cancer death in American men. For the year 2008, it was projected that 186,000 men would be diagnosed and that 28,700 deaths would occur from prostate cancer (Jemal et al. 2008). The increasing incidence of prostate cancer and the morbidity and mortality of the disease and its treatments, combined with an improved insight into its biologic basis and hormone dependency, have led to a focus on chemoprevention strategies.

Chemoprevention refers to the use of therapeutic agents to prevent cancer or the adverse outcomes of cancer. Multiple factors, including high incidence, long latency period between initial evidence of prostate cancer and the development of overt or lethal disease, and advanced age of onset (Gronberg 2003; Majeed et al. 2000), make prostate cancer an ideal target for chemoprevention strategies. Even a modest delay in development of symptomatic cancer may be sufficient to reduce the incidence of the disease, improve survival, and prevent the complications of the disease and the morbidities of its treatments.

H.-J. Senn and F. Otto (eds.), *Clinical Cancer Prevention*,
Recent Results in Cancer Research 188, DOI: 10.1007/978-3-642-10858-7_9,

9

9.2 The Prostate Cancer Prevention Trial

The goal of the PCPT was to test the hypothesis that finasteride could prevent prostate cancer. A total of 18, 822 men, at least 55 years of age, with a normal digital rectal examination (DRE) and a baseline prostate-specific antigen (PSA) level less than 3 ng/mL, were enrolled and randomly assigned to finasteride (5 mg/day) or placebo for 7 years. Prostate biopsy was recommended if the subsequent annual PSA level, adjusted for the finasteride effect (the adjustment factor of 2–2.5) (Etzioni et al. 2005), exceeded 4 ng/mL or if a DRE was suspicious. The primary endpoint of the study was the prevalence of prostate cancer diagnosed by "for-cause" biopsies or "end-of-study" biopsies during the 7 years of study. The PCPT reported that there was a 24.8% reduction in the incidence of prostate cancer from 24.4% with placebo to 18.4% in men treated with finasteride. The authors also noted that the magnitude of the risk reduction did not differ according to PSA level, age, race/ethnicity, or family history of prostate cancer (Thompson et al. 2003).

The PCPT trial also reported that high-grade tumors of Gleason grade 7–10 were more common in the finasteride group than in the placebo group. This apparent increase in the incidence of high-grade prostate cancer resulted in a general lack of acceptance of finasteride for prostate cancer prevention. Subsequent analyses yielded additional information that resulted in an observed overall risk reduction of 27% (Redman et al. 2008).

9.3 Pathologic Characteristics of the Cancers in the Prostate Cancer Prevention Trial

A major concern about early detection of prostate cancer by PSA and prevention by finasteride is the discovery of and responsibility to treat biologically inconsequential tumors that would otherwise remain undetected during a man's lifetime in the absence of screening or aggressive biopsy strategies or both. The established pathologic definition of a clinically insignificant tumor is an organ-confined, low-volume, and low-Gleason score tumor (Epstein et al. 1994). The most commonly cited criteria for insignificant disease on biopsy proposed by Epstein et al. (1994) are a combination of clinical factors (stage T1c and PSA density <0.15 ng/mL/g), grade of tumor (Gleason score ≤6, with no Gleason 4 or 5), and extent of tumor (<3 cores with tumor [no core with >50% tumor] or <3 mm cancer present in only one core).

Lucia et al. (2008) reviewed the pathologic characteristics of prostate biopsies from men in the placebo and finasteride groups of the PCPT. These authors found that 75% of all cancers and 62% of Gleason score 6 or less cancers met the biopsy criteria for clinically significant tumors. In addition, surrogate measures for tumor volume, including volume of disease on biopsy, and risk of perineural invasion were lower in men who received finasteride. The PSA-associated risks of insignificant cancer were 51.7% (PSA 0–1.0 ng/mL), 33.7% (1.1–2.5 ng/mL), 17.8% (2.6–4 ng/mL), and 11.7% (4.1–10 ng/mL). Conversely, the risks of high-grade tumors for the same PSA strata were 15.6, 37.9, 49.1, and 52.4%, respectively. This study revealed that approximately only 25% of detected tumors met the criteria for insignificance, a rate similar to the findings of the contemporary series of men who undergo treatment for their disease (Epstein et al. 1998). This analysis suggests that men who developed prostate cancer on finasteride had a lower tumor volume and decrease in aggressive features across all tumor grades as compared with those in the placebo arm. About two-thirds of all detected tumors and half of Gleason score 6 or less, which finasteride is known to prevent, met the definition for clinical significance. Tumors among men treated with finasteride were small and had less extensive characteristics.

Lucia et al. (2007) assessed whether the increased high-grade prostate cancer associated with finasteride in the PCPT was due to finasteride's potential effects on tumor morphology or prostate size and found that effects on volume and selective inhibition of low-grade cancer may have contributed to the original PCPT findings. Prostate biopsies with Gleason score 8–10 were examined histologically for hormonal effects and those with Gleason score 7–10 were examined for pathologic surrogates of disease extent. Prostate volumes were measured at biopsy. Samples from radical prostatectomy (n = 222, finasteride; n = 306, placebo) were examined for tumor grade and extent. Grades at biopsy and prostatectomy were compared between the groups. They found that prostate volumes were lower in the finasteride group at 25.1 versus 34.4 cm^3 and that pathologic surrogates for tumor aggressiveness were lower with finasteride than with placebo. Among patients who had a prostatectomy, the finasteride-associated increase in high-grade disease at biopsy was diminished at prostatectomy. However, in the finasteride group, biopsy identified a greater proportion of patients with high-grade disease present at prostatectomy. These results suggest that high-grade cancer was detected earlier and was less extensive in the finasteride group than in the placebo group.

9.4 Finasteride Increases Sensitivity of Prostate-Specific Antigen, Digital Rectal Examination and Biopsy Detection for Prostate Cancer

Observations made after the PCPT suggested that the increase in high-grade disease in the finasteride group may have been secondary to detection bias rather than an actual alteration in the natural history of the disease (Thompson et al. 2003). In 2006, Thompson et al. (2006) examined the impact of finasteride on the sensitivity and area under the receiver operating characteristics curve (AUC) of PSA for detecting prostate cancer. They compared the placebo and finasteride groups for sensitivity and AUC of PSA for the detection of all cancers and for high-grade cancers. The AUC of PSA for all outcomes was greater for the finasteride group than the placebo group. The sensitivity of PSA was higher for men in the finasteride group than in the placebo group at all PSA cutoffs matched by specificity.

When the PCPT was designed, the authors hypothesized that finasteride could influence the detection of prostate cancer by decreasing the size of the prostate, making the DRE more sensitive. To investigate this theory, Thompson et al. (2007) again published a repeat analysis of the PCPT data in 2007. They examined the sensitivity and specificity of DRE in the finasteride and placebo groups in patients who had a biopsy, PSA measurement, and DRE within 1 year before the biopsy, and were on treatment at the time of biopsy. They found that the sensitivity of DRE was significantly greater for cancer detection in men receiving finasteride than placebo (21.3 versus 16.7%, P = 0.015). In addition, although it did not attain statistical significance, DRE sensitivity was greater for detecting high-grade cancers in men on finasteride.

Since the original publication of the PCPT data, we now know that finasteride enhances the detection of prostate cancer on "for-cause" biopsies by improved sensitivity of PSA for overall and high-grade cancer detection (Thompson et al. 2006; Ankerst and Thompson 2006), improved sensitivity of DRE (Thompson et al. 2007), increased sensitivity of biopsy for high-grade cancer detection (Cohen et al. 2007), and more accurate grading of high-grade prostate cancer (Lucia et al. 2007; Thompson et al. 2006; Scardino 2003).

A recently performed series of analyses (Redman et al. 2008) systematically controlled these and other factors in estimating the true rate of cancer in the two study groups of the PCPT.

9

They incorporated adjustments for all of the aforementioned biases and showed that the cancer detection rates on biopsy in the entire PCPT of 15,990 men would have been similar, though slightly lower, than were observed in the 10,182 men who actually had an endpoint determinate. Estimated overall prostate cancer rates were 14.7% (4.8% high grade) for finasteride and 21.1% (4.2% high grade) for placebo, a 30% risk reduction in prostate cancer and a nonsignificant 14% increase in high-grade cancer with finasteride. Next, they extended to the entire PCPT population the changes from biopsy grade to prostatectomy grade, using data from the subset of 500 men who had a prostatectomy. The resulting rates, or "true" rates, of high-grade disease were 8.2% in the placebo arm and 6.0% in the finasteride arm, resulting in a 27% relative risk reduction in high-grade disease in the finasteride arm. This suggests that it was highly unlikely that finasteride actually increased the risk of high-grade cancer in the PCPT.

The third analysis examined the impact of biopsy sensitivity on the relative risk of high-grade prostate cancer and found that differential sensitivity of biopsy between the treatment arms can have a significant impact on risk ratio estimates. Biopsy sensitivity for high-grade disease is known to be lower with placebo than with finasteride, as has been shown previously (Lucia et al. 2007). Different ranges of biopsy sensitivity for high-grade cancer resulted in either a null or a reduced relative risk in the finasteride group for high-grade cancer. This final analysis revealed that as the sensitivity of prostate biopsy improves with finasteride, an even larger reduction in high-grade tumors is observed. This explains how small differences in biopsy sensitivity between the study arms could result in the apparent finasteride-associated increase in high grades on biopsy that was reported in 2003 (Thompson et al. 2003).

Overall, this study suggests that the originally observed higher risk of high-grade cancer with finasteride seems to have been due to facilitated diagnosis resulting primarily from increased biopsy sensitivity and that finasteride can actually reduce the risk of all prostate cancers, regardless of grade (Redman et al. 2008).

9.4.1 Decreased Prostate Volume with Finasteride Increases Cancer Detection

Despite reduction in the total number of prostate cancers in the PCPT, the originally observed increase in the number of patients with high-grade cancer dramatically weakened interest in the use of finasteride as a chemopreventive agent (Unger et al. 2003; Grover et al. 2006; Zeliadt et al. 2005; Andriole et al. 2007). One theory speculated that there were more high-grade tumors identified due to an alteration in the histological appearance of the tumor due to finasteride effects. As previously discussed, review of the specimens from the PCPT did not support this theory and revealed that finasteride did not affect the Gleason grade (Lucia et al. 2007).

Further analyses indicated that the effect of finasteride on normal prostate and on low-grade prostate cancer led to biases favoring the diagnosis of high-grade disease in men treated with finasteride (Redman et al. 2008; Lucia et al. 2008; Cohen et al. 2007; Pinsky et al. 2008). This was illustrated by a reanalysis of the PCPT results that supported a diagnostic bias due to the effect of finasteride on prostate size (Cohen et al. 2007). Patients treated with finasteride had a significantly smaller prostate volume (median 25.1 versus 33.5 cm^3 with placebo). The conclusion from this article is that the reduction in prostate volume with finasteride results in a disproportionate sampling of the tumor during biopsy, thereby increasing identification of high-grade tumor. When the effect of prostate size was incorporated into the analysis, the increased risk of high-grade prostate cancer with finasteride disappeared as compared with placebo. These results provide further reassurance that finasteride does not result in a clinically relevant increase in the number of high-grade prostate cancers (Cohen et al. 2007).

9.5 Side Effects of Finasteride

Sexual dysfunction was a prespecified secondary endpoint of the PCPT because of its large study population and long follow-up period. The results of this analysis demonstrated that finasteride had only a modest affect on sexual function and its impact diminished over time (Moinpour et al. 2007). The increase in the Sexual Activity Scale score (on a scale of 0–100) relative to placebo of 3.21 points at the first assessment decreased to 2.11 points at the end of study. After adjustment for all covariates, mean sexual dysfunction increased in both arms from baseline (6 months after randomization) by 1.26 Sexual Activity points per year, corresponding to a cumulative increase of 8.22 points. Men on finasteride had an average score of 3.21 points higher than men on placebo but the effect diminished with time. This study reveals that sexual dysfunction with finasteride is not clinically significant and should minimally influence the decision to treat with finasteride (Sarvis and Thompson 2008).

9.6 Conclusion

The decision of whether or not to use finasteride in individual cases requires an informed decision that balances the potential benefits of finasteride against the known potential side effects of prolonged treatment. Patients must weigh the established benefits of a 25–30% reduction in prostate cancer, decreased urinary symptoms, and decreased complications of an enlarged prostate against the established side effects, which include clinically insignificant reduced sexual function and expense of medication.

We find no evidence that finasteride increased the risk of high-grade prostate cancer in the PCPT. Therefore, we conclude that men who are 55 years of age or older need not be concerned about an increased risk of high-grade prostate cancer with finasteride. With an excellent safety profile and minimal side effects, men aged 55 years or older should be informed of the opportunity to reduce their risk of prostate cancer with finasteride. We conclude that the promise of prostate cancer prevention is a reality and that the findings of the PCPT provide the momentum and foundation for further studies into chemopreventive agents.

References

Andriole G, Bostwick D, Brawley O et al (2004) Chemoprevention of prostate cancer in men at high risk: rationale and design of the Reduction by Dutasteride of Prostate Cancer Events (REDUCE) trial. J Urol 172(4 Pt 1):1314–1317

Andriole GL, Humphrey PA, Serfling RJ, Grubb RL (2007) High-grade prostate cancer in the Prostate Cancer Prevention trial: fact or artifact? J Natl Cancer Inst 99:1355–1356

Ankerst DP, Thompson IM (2006) Sensitivity and specificity of prostate-specific antigen for prostate cancer detection with high rates of biopsy verification. Arch Ital Urol Androl 78:125–129

Clark RV, Hermann DJ, Cunningham GR et al (2004) Marked suppression of dihydrotestosterone in men with benign prostatic hyperplasia by dutasteride, a dual 5 alpha-reductase inhibitor. J Clin Endocrinol Metab 89:2179–2184

Cohen YC, Liu KS, Heyden NL et al (2007) Detection bias due to the effect of finasteride on prostate volume: a modeling approach for analysis of the Prostate Cancer Prevention trial. J Natl Cancer Inst 99:1366–1374, Patients treated with finasteride had a significantly smaller prostate volume resulting in a disproportionate sampling of the tumor during biopsy, allowing for increased identification of high-grade tumor

9

Epstein JI, Walsh PC, Carmichael M, Brendler CB (1994) Pathologic and clinical findings to predict tumor extent of nonpalpable (stage T1c) prostate cancer. JAMA 271:368–374

Epstein JI, Chan DW, Sokoll LJ et al (1998) Nonpalpable stage T1c prostate cancer: prediction of insignificant disease using free/total prostate specific antigen levels and needle biopsy findings. J Urol 160(6 Pt 2):2407–2411

Etzioni RD, Howlader N, Shaw PA et al (2005) Long-term effects of finasteride on prostate specific antigen levels: results from the Prostate Cancer Prevention trial. J Urol 174:877–881

Gronberg H (2003) Prostate cancer epidemiology. Lancet 361:859–864

Grover S, Lowensteyn I, Hajek D et al (2006) Do the benefits of finasteride outweigh the risks in the Prostate Cancer Prevention trial? J Urol 175(3 Pt 1) :934–938, discussion 938 [Context Link]

Jemal A, Siegel R, Ward E et al (2008) Cancer statistics, 2008. CA Cancer J Clin 58:71–96

Lucia MS, Epstein JI, Goodman PJ et al (2007) Finasteride and high-grade prostate cancer in the Prostate Cancer Prevention trial. J Natl Cancer Inst 99:1375–1383, Prostate volumes were lower and pathologic surrogates for tumor aggressiveness were lower with finasteride than with placebo. These results suggest that high-grade cancer was detected earlier and was less extensive in the finasteride group than in the placebo group

Lucia MS, Darke AK, Goodman PJ et al (2008) Pathologic characteristics of cancers detected in the Prostate Cancer Prevention trial: implications for prostate cancer detection and chemoprevention. Cancer Prev Res 1:167–173, Men who developed prostate cancer on finasteride had a lower tumor volume and less aggressive disease across all tumor grades as compared with those in placebo arm

Majeed A, Babb P, Jones J, Quinn M (2000) Trends in prostate cancer incidence, mortality and survival in England and Wales 1971–1998. BJU Int 85:1058–1062

McConnell JD, Wilson JD, George FW et al (1992) Finasteride, an inhibitor of 5 alpha-reductase, suppresses prostatic dihydrotestosterone in men with benign prostatic hyperplasia. J Clin Endocrinol Metab 74:505–508

Moinpour CM, Darke AK, Donaldson GW et al (2007) Longitudinal analysis of sexual function reported by men in the Prostate Cancer Prevention trial. J Natl Cancer Inst 99:1025–1035, Finasteride had only a modest affect on sexual function and its impact diminished over time [Context Link]

Pinsky P, Parnes HL, Ford L (2008) Estimating rates of true high-grade disease in the Prostate Cancer Prevention trial. Cancer Prev Res 1:182–186 [Context Link]

Redman MW, Tangen C, Goodman P et al (2008) Finasteride does not increase the risk of high-grade prostate cancer: a bias-adjusted modeling approach. Cancer Prev Res 1:174–181, Finasteride does not cause high-grade prostate cancer and reduces the risk of high-grade tumors by 27% and reduces the risk of low-grade tumors by 34%

Scardino PT (2003) The prevention of prostate cancer – the dilemma continues. N Engl J Med 349:297–299

Thompson IM () Prostate cancer chemoprevention: update of the Prostate Cancer Prevention trial findings and implications for clinical practice. Curr Oncol Rep 10:529–532

Thompson IM, Goodman PJ, Tangen CM et al (2003) The influence of finasteride on the development of prostate cancer. N Engl J Med 349:215–224

Thompson IM, Chi C, Ankerst DP et al (2006) Effect of finasteride on the sensitivity of PSA for detecting prostate cancer. J Natl Cancer Inst 98:1128–1133

Thompson IM, Tangen CM, Goodman PJ et al (2007) Finasteride improves the sensitivity of digital rectal examination for prostate cancer detection. J Urol 177:1749–1752, The sensitivity of DRE was significantly greater for cancer detection in men receiving finasteride than placebo (21.3 versus 16.7%, P = 0.015)

Unger JM, LeBlanc M, Crowley JJ et al (2003) Estimating the impact of new clinical trial proven cancer therapy and cancer chemoprevention on population mortality: the Karnofsky Memorial lecture. J Clin Oncol 21(23 Suppl):246–252

Zeliadt SB, Etzioni RD, Penson DF et al (2005) Lifetime implications and cost-effectiveness of using finasteride to prevent prostate cancer. Am J Med 118:850–857

10 Hormone Replacement Therapy and Breast Cancer

Anthony Howell and Gareth D. Evans

Abstract There is evidence that hormone replacement therapy (HRT) may both stimulate and inhibit breast cancers, giving rise to a spectrum of activities, which are frequently hard to understand. Here we summarise the evidence for these paradoxical effects and, given the current data, attempt to give an indication where it may or may not be appropriate to prescribe HRT.

It is clear that administration of oestrogen-progestin (E-P) and oestrogen alone (E) HRT is sufficient to stimulate the growth of overt breast tumours in women since withdrawal of HRT results in reduction of proliferation of primary tumours and withdrawal responses in metastatic tumours. E-P, E including tibolone are associated with increased local and distant relapse when given after surgery for breast cancer. For women given HRT who do not have breast cancer the only large randomised trial (WHI) of E-P or E versus placebo has produced some expected and also paradoxical results. E-P increases breast cancer risk as previously shown in observational studies. Risk is increased, particularly in women known to be compliant. Conversely, E either has no effect or reduces breast cancer risk consistent with some but not all observational studies. Two observational studies report a decrease or at least no increase in risk when E-P or E are given after oophorectomy in young women with *BRCA1/2* mutations. Early oophorectomy increases death rates from cardiovascular and other conditions and there is evidence that this may be reversed by the use of E post-oophorectomy. HRT may thus reduce the risk of breast cancer and other diseases (e.g., cardiovascular) in young women and increase or decrease them in older women.

10.1 Background

After the discovery of oestrogens (Allen and Doisy 1923), hormone replacement therapy (HRT) was introduced in the 1930s. Conjugated equine estrogens (CEE) were licensed by the American Food and Drug Administration in 1942. However, concern was raised after the use of oestrogen only HRT because of the increased risk of endometrial cancer (Smith et al. 1975). The reported excess risk was 4.5-fold although the increase was not seen until after 5 years of use. The excess risk of endometrial cancer was solved by adding a progestogen to E, but it soon became apparent from observational studies

A. Howell (✉) and G.D. Evans
Genesis Prevention Centre, University Hospital of South Manchester, Manchester, M23 9LT, UK
e-mail: anthony.howell@christie.nhs.uk

H.-J. Senn and F. Otto (eds.), *Clinical Cancer Prevention*,
Recent Results in Cancer Research 188, DOI: 10.1007/978-3-642-10858-7_10,

that, not only was E alone associated with increased breast cancer risk, but that the magnitude of this risk appeared greater in women using E+P (Hoover et al. 1976; Bergkvist et al. 1989). A re-analysis of all HRT studies by the Collaborative Group on Hormonal Factors in Breast Cancer (1997) of 51 epidemiological studies in 52,705 women with breast cancer and 108,411 controls without breast cancer reported in 1987 indicated a relative risk of 1.35 (95% CI 1.21–1.49; 2 $p=0.00001$) for women who used HRT for 5 years or longer. This overview of the available data from observational studies was followed by a single observational study which recruited over one million women already undergoing mammographic screening in the UK National Breast Screening Programme (The Million Women Study, Beral 2003). Current users of HRT at recruitment were more likely than never users to develop breast cancer (RR 1.66, 95% CI 1.58–1.75, $p<0001$]). This was the first study to indicate increased breast cancer deaths in women using HRT (RR 1.22 95%CI 1.00–1.48, $p=0.05$). Past users of HRT were not at an increased risk of or death from breast cancer. The first of the Women's Health Initiative (WHI) randomised trials, which compared CEE and medroxyprogesterone acetate (MPA), was reported in 2002 (Rossouw et al. 2002). After a mean of 5.2 years of follow-up, there was increased risk of breast cancer in E+P users (RR 1.26, 95% CI1.00–1.59). The publication of the results of the WHI study produced a marked decline in the use of HRT and also the incidence of breast cancer first reported by Ravdin et al. in 2007. The CEE v placebo WHI trial later showed that up to 7 years use of CEE was associated with a non-significant decrease in breast cancer risk (WHI Steering Committee 2004). A later randomised study using tibolone showed a reduced risk (Cummings et al. 2008). Observational studies demonstrated that HRT reduced the risk of recurrence of breast cancer when given after surgery (Col et al. 2005), but two randomised trials indicated an increased risk of recurrence, one where E or E+P used according to clinical indication was compared with no HRT (Holmberg et al. 2008) and the other using tibolone compared with placebo (Kenemans et al. 2009). In this review we will summarise the results of HRT in relation to the growth of diagnosed breast cancer and also risk of breast cancer in women above and below the age of 50 treated with HRT. We include observational studies and randomised trials and highlight the fact that the results of the two types of study often produce divergent results.

10.2 HRT Use in Women Diagnosed with Breast Cancer

10.2.1 Observational Studies

As noted above, Col et al. reported an overview of eight observational studies assessing the effect of giving HRT to women after surgery for breast cancer for the relief of symptoms. Only studies that included patients with invasive breast cancer who received oral HRT, that had an explicitly defined comparison group, and that reported breast cancer recurrences were included. The eight studies involved a total of 3,710 patients with a mean age of 59.7 years, a mean disease-free interval of 49.2 months, duration of HRT use of 28 months, and a mean follow-up period after HRT initiation of 57.1 months. A combined total of 552 recurrences (109 among HRT users) and 460 deaths (51 among HRT users) occurred in these trials. The pooled RR for the observational studies was 0.64 (95% CI 0.50–0.82). Prognostic factors for HRT users and non-users differed in most studies. On average, HRT users were more than 3 years younger than non-users and were more likely to be node negative. Because these studies demonstrated that HRT was not only of symptomatic benefit to women after surgery but also indicated an actual reduction of breast cancer risk, these were of great importance to the management of women after surgery and it was felt that they should be confirmed by appropriately designed randomised trials.

10.2.2 Randomised Trials

Four randomised trials have been reported. The first entered only 100 patients and had to be abandoned (Marsden et al. 2000). In the Stockholm Trial (Von Schoultz et al. 2005) 378 patients were randomised between no treatment or HRT (E or E+P as clinically indicated). There were no statistical differences in the rate of relapse between the use of hormone therapy or not. However, two other trials showed an increased risk of breast cancer relapse after surgery in women randomised to HRT. In the HABITS study (Holmberg et al. 2008) 442 women were randomly assigned to treatment with E or E+P as clinically indicated versus no additional treatment. Thirty-nine of the 221 women in the HRT arm and 17 of the 221 women in the control arm experienced a new breast cancer event (RR 2.4, 95% CI 1.3–4.2). The incidence of relapse at 5 years was 22.2% in the HRT arm and 8.0% in the control arm. Increased risk was seen in women with node positive and negative tumours, whether treated with adjuvant tamoxifen or not. There were no differences in the numbers of deaths from breast cancer. In 2002, the organisers of the HABITS and Stockholm trials agreed to pool safety analyses and to use a joint IDMSC. In October 2003, the combined estimate of the hazard ratio (HR) for recurrence with HRT compared with recurrence without HRT reached 1.8 (95% CI = 1.03 to 3.1) and was thus statistically significantly larger than 1.0, and the trials were stopped in 2003. The third trial (LIBERATE) was a randomisation between 2.6 mg of tibolone daily or placebo (Kenemans et al. 2009). There were 1,556 patients in the tibolone arm and 1,542 patients in the placebo arm of the trial. Treatment was initiated at a mean of 2.1 years after surgery. After a median follow-up of 3.1 years, 15.2% of women randomised to tibolone had a cancer recurrence compared with 10.7% of patients randomised to placebo (RR 1.4, 95% CI 1.14–1.70; $p=0.001$). There was no significant effect of tibolone on the risk of relapse in women with ER–ve tumours (Kenemans et al. 2009).

It is not clear why the Stockholm trial result differed but the balance of evidence suggests that it is detrimental to use HRT on women with ER+ve breast cancer but, perhaps could be used cautiously in women with ER–ve tumours.

10.2.3 Effects of Withdrawal of HRT in Women with Breast Cancer

Another indication of the promotional effect of HRT on breast cancer is to assess what happens after the withdrawal of treatment with HRT Howell A (1992). Two studies of women taking HRT showed that there was evidence of regression of overt breast cancer when the HRT was stopped. Dhodapkar et al. (1995) reported three women who had been given CEE some years after surgery for breast cancer. The women were taking CEE from between 5 and 17 years after surgery, relapsed whilst taking HRT in the lung, the bones or both sites. The only treatment given was to stop the HRT at the time of relapse and all three women had a response to withdrawing the CEE they were taking and the response lasted 3 years in all three cases. A further patient presenting with metastatic breast cancer whilst taking CEE also had a regression after the CEE was stopped. In all four cases the withdrawal response indicates that the relapse was stimulated by CEE.

10

In a second study, Prasad et al. (2003) reported the effect of withdrawing HRT at the time a primary tumour is detected on proliferation of the tumour. A biopsy of the breast was taken at presentation and at a median of 17 days later when definitive surgery was performed. Women who stopped HRT had a significant decrease in Ki67 expression but only if their tumour was oestrogen receptor positive (ER+ve) (n = 106, $p<0.001$). No change in proliferation was seen in women who continued HRT up until the time of surgery. The observed reduction of proliferation or growth after relapse indicates that in overt breast cancer HRT is associated with stimulation of growth.

10.3 HRT and Risk of Breast Cancer

10.3.1 Observational Studies

The major observational studies of the Collaborative Group on Hormonal Factors and Breast Cancer (1997) and the Million Women Study (Beral and Million Women Study 2003) indicate that E-P, E and tibolone increase the risk of breast cancer. The overview of all HRT studies by the Collaborative Group (1997) was of 51 epidemiological studies in 52,705 women with breast cancer and 108,411 women without breast cancer and indicated a relative risk of 1.35 (95% CI 1.21–1.49; 2 $p=0.00001$) for women who had used HRT for 5 years or longer. In the Million Women Study, incidence was significantly increased for current users of preparations containing E only (HR1.30, 95% CI 1.21–1.40, $p<0.001$) and E+P (HR 2.00, 95% CI1.88–2.12, $p<0.001$). In this study, tibolone was also associated with increased breast cancer risk (HR1.45, 95% CI1.25–1.68, $p < 0001$). Results varied little between specific types of estrogens and progestogens or their doses (or between continuous and sequential regimens of E+P).

10.3.2 Randomised Studies

The WHI randomised trial of placebo (8,102 women between the ages of 50 and 74) versus CEE 0.625 mg/day and MPA 2.5 mg/day (8,506 women) was initiated in 1993 and stopped after a mean of 5.2 years of follow-up. There was an increased risk of breast cancer (1.24 95% CI 1.02–1.50), significantly increased risks of cardiovascular disease (CHD), stroke and pulmonary embolism and significantly decreased risks of hip fracture and colorectal cancer (Rossouw et al. 2002, 2007; Chlebowski et al. 2003). The curves for breast cancer were comparable for the first 4 years but separated thereafter in the overall analysis and at 3 years in adherent women. There was no increased risk in women who had no prior HRT use (HR 1.06 95% CI 0.81–1.38). However there was evidence of a positive trend in HR in years from randomisation in the trial overall in the prior and no-prior E+P groups. A separate analysis of the prior and no-prior E+P groups indicated an increased risk in the no-prior group after about 5 years of follow-up (Anderson et al. 2006). Over one third of the women stopped study medication. When women who were non-compliant were censored 6 months after stopping study medication the HR for breast cancer in the compliant group rose to 1.49 (95% CI 1.13–1.96-Weighted $p<0.001$). The risks of breast cancer were not significantly higher in women with a family history or other risk factors. Although they were of similar grade, tumours arising on E+P were likely to be larger and node positive, possibly related to the effect of E+P on mammographic density obscuring detection by mammography (Chlebowski et al. 2003). There were no differences in the ratio of ER+ versus ER–ve cancers.

In the WHI randomised comparison of CEE (0.625 mg/day n=5310 women) and placebo (n = 5429 women) in women aged 50–79 years there was a non-significant decrease in risk of invasive breast cancer (HR 0.80 95%CI 0.62–1.04 $p=0.09$) after a mean follow up of 7.1 years.

In a sensitivity analysis, when women who were less than 80% compliant with medication were censored 6 months after last use, there was a significant reduction in breast cancer risk (HR 0.67 95% CI 0.47–0.97 $p=0.03$, Stefanick et al. 2006) and in women with no prior hormonal use (No prior use HR 0.65 95% CI 0.46–0.92. Prior use HR 1.02 95% CI 0.70–1.50). Invasive breast cancers were larger compared with placebo (1.8 v 1.5 cm $p<0.30$) and a higher proportion tended to be node positive (35.5% v 23.3% respectively $p<0.07$). Analyses suggest that the decreased risk was related to a reduction in localised disease, invasive duct (and not lobular cancers) and was not reduced in women with a family history of breast cancer. Tibolone is a form of HRT which has oestrogenic, androgenic and progestogenic effects. In a randomised trial of 4,538 women aged between 60 and 85 years after a median of 34 months of treatment the tibolone group had a decreased risk of invasive breast cancer (HR 0.32 95% CI 0.13–0.80 $p=0.03$).

10.3.3 Withdrawal of HRT in Women Without Breast Cancer

After the Women's Health Initiative studies, there was a marked decline in the use of HRT in the United States and many other countries. This reduction in use of HRT was associated with a decrease in the annual age-adjusted incidence of 8.6% in the United States (Ravdin et al. 2007). Decrease was seen mainly in cancers that were ER positive. In Australia, prescriptions for HRT increased from 1996 to 2001 but dropped by 40% from 2001 to 2003 (Canfell et al. 2008). The age standardised breast cancer incidence rates in women increased to 2001 but declined thereafter. The incidence in women of 50 years of age or above was lower by 6.7% in 2003 compared with 2001. The decline in incidence of breast cancer was also reported in the California Teachers Study cohort (Marshall et al. 2010). The strength of this study was that women were mailed to determine their HRT usage. This group reported a significant decline of breast cancer by 26% in women between the dates 2000–2002 and 2003–2005. The decline in invasive breast cancer incidence rates was restricted to oestrogen receptor positive tumours. The decline was seen after E=P or E was stopped. During this period the incidence of breast cancer did not change significantly for women who never took HRT.

10.3.4 Summary

Thus, observational studies indicate that E+P, E (including tibolone) produce an increase in risk of breast cancer. The WHI randomised studies were in agreement with observational studies with respect to E+P, but they demonstrated no increase at least in the short term of about 7 years of CEE alone. Also the Million Women Study demonstrated an increase in risk of tibolone, whereas a randomised trial of tibolone versus placebo in women with osteoporosis showed a reduction in risk in women prescribed tibolone (Cummings et al. 2008). However, the studies cited that, particularly the California Teachers Study cohort, there was a reduction on both women who were taking E and E+P. Thus, although there is no increase in risk on CEE in the short term in WHI, other studies show that longer-term use of CEE is associated with increased risk and thus this presumably explains the reduction on risk in E alone as well as E+P after withdrawal of HRT (Chen et al. 2006).

10.4 HRT After Oophorectomy in Women Less Than 50 Years of Age

The studies outlined above were performed mainly in women above the age of 50 and did not have sufficient data to report separately in younger women. However, many women have oophorectomy before the age of 50 and others have an early natural menopause. This is particularly seen in women with *BRCA1* and *BRCA2* mutations since early oophorectomy reduces the risk of both breast and ovarian cancer (Domchek et al. 2006; Kurian et al. 2010). The question arises whether it is safe to administer HRT in women under the age of 50, particularly in those with an increased risk of breast cancer related to mutations in breast cancer predisposing genes.

10.4.1 Observational Studies

It is not possible to randomise mutation carriers to HRT versus not, but two observational studies suggest that HRT use is not associated with increased risk of the development of breast cancer after oophorectomy in carriers. Rebbeck et al. (2005) studied a cohort of 462 women with germline *BRCA1/2* mutations at 13 medical centres to evaluate breast cancer risk after oophorectomy with and without HRT. HRT of any type did not significantly alter the reduction in breast cancer risk after oophorectomy (0.40, 0.18–0.92 without HRT and 0.37, 0.14–0.96 with HRT). Eisen et al. (2008) performed a matched case control study in 472 postmenopausal women with mutations in the *BRCA1* gene. Women who developed breast cancer were matched with respect to age, age at menopause and type of menopause. The adjusted odds ratios for breast cancer associated with ever use of HRT compared with never use was 0.58 (95% CI 0.35–0.96 $p=0.03$), however the association with the use of E+P was not statistically significant (OR=0.51 95% CI 0.27–0.98 $p=0.21$). The OR did not depend on the age of diagnosis or the age of menopause and there was no apparent modification of the OR by duration of use and similar for current and past users.

In the general population of women, a Danish cohort study suggested a non-significant decrease in risk of breast cancer in women given HRT below the age of 50 (Ewertz et al. 2005). These investigators examined the risk of developing breast cancer in relation to HRT (by examining numbers of HRT prescriptions) in a cohort of 78,380 women aged 40–67 years from 1989–2002. A total of 1,462 cases of breast cancers were identified during a mean follow-up of 10 years. In women between the ages of 40 and 44 the RR of breast cancer was 0.56 (95% CI 0.07–2.01) and in the group aged 45 and 49 the RR was 0.88 (95% CI 0.62–1.22). Restricting the cohort to women aged 50 years or more at entry, an increased risk associated with current use of HRT was seen as reported in other observational studies in women of this age (RR1.61, 95% CI1.38–1.88). The risk increased with duration of use; no material risk difference was observed amongst various HRT regimens. Thus, these limited data outlined above in women under 50 suggest either no difference in risk or reduction in risk in mutation carriers and in the general population.

10.5 Coronary Heart Disease

In the first report from the WHI (Rossouw et al. 2002) of the results of E+P use after a median of 4.2 years, there was a significant increased risk of CHD (HR 1.29 95%CI 1.02–1.63). CHD was defined as non-fatal myocardial infarction and CHD death. The absolute excess risk was seven more CHD events per 10,000 years. These data, together with the significant excess of breast cancers after 4 years' use and the increased risk of stroke and thrombo-embolic disease associated with HRT, triggered the stopping of the trial after a median follow-up of 5.2 years. In the E alone study there was a non-significant decrease in CHD overall (WHI Steering Committee 2004).

The results of the E+P and E for CHD with respect to age were reported separately by

Roussouw et al. in 2007. In women aged 50–59 years of age at entry to the E+P trial there was a non-significant increase in CHD (HR 1.29 (%% CI 0.79–2.12) and stroke (HR 1.41 95% CI 0.75) and a non-significant decrease in total mortality (HR 0.69 95% CI 0.44–1.07). In women 50–59 years of age at entry into the E alone trial there were non-significant reduction of CHD (HR 0.63 95% CI 0.36–1.09), stroke (HR 0.89 95% CI 0.47–1.69) and total mortality (RH 0.71 95% CI 0.46–1.11). The figures were similar for women within 10 years of the menopause

The data outlined above indicate that there is no significant increase in CHD in younger women in the trial. However, there is evidence that that an early menopause, whether natural or induced, is associated with reduced life expectancy, mainly from CVD but also other diseases (Dubey et al. 2005; Lobo 2007). An increase in mortality was seen in a long-term observational study in Minnesota, USA. From 1950 to 1957 mortality associated with cardiovascular disease was assessed in 1,274 women with unilateral oophorectomy compared with 1,091 women with bilateral oophorectomy in comparison with 2,383 referent women in the same population. Women who underwent bilateral oophorectomy before the age 45 experienced an increased mortality associated with CHD compared with referent women (1.44, 1.01–2.05, $p=0.04$). Mortality was significantly increased in women who were not treated with E though aged 45 but not in women treated with E (Rivera et al. 2009). An increased mortality after oophorectomy before age 50 was also demonstrated in the Nurses Health Study. After over 24 years of follow-up, women with hysterectomy and bilateral oophorectomy were compared with ovarian conservation: multivariable hazard ratios were 1.12 (1.03–1.21) for total mortality and 1.17 (1.02–1.35) for fatal and non-fatal cardiovascular disease (Parker et al. 2009). In a decision analysis model for women with *BRCA1* and *BRCA2* mutations, oophorectomy at age 40 was associated with increased life expectancy and this was further increased in women given E (Kurian et al. 2010) .

Thus in the WHI trials there was no increase in CHD risk in women between age 50 and 59 (although there was an increase in stroke and thromboembolic disease). In younger women an early menopause increases CHD and decreases mortality, which may be reversed by E.

10.6 Potential Biological Explanations

We have summarised data with respect to breast cancer, CHD and mortality for HRT use after surgery and in women in the general population Often many observational data are in complete disagreement with data derived from clinical trials and we will focus on the results of trial data if available. The increased relapse after surgery induced by E+P, E and tibolone are consistent with the known stimulatory effects of E and P on breast tumours and the normal breast. The fact that recurrence is stimulated in women with ER+ve tumours and withdrawal responses occur after cessation of HRT is consistent with a stimulatory effect. It is more difficult to explain the reduction of risk of breast cancer with E (WHI) and tibolone (LIFT trial). However, in pre-clinical models, breast cancer of cells in vitro (Liu et al. 2003; Song et al. 2001) and breast cancer xenografts (Lewis et al. 2005; Bernstein et al. 2004) demonstrate apoptosis or tumour regression in response to low-dose oestrogen. Thus E may change from being stimulatory to inhibitory depending on timing and the hormonal environment. This is consistent with tamoxifen changing from an antagonist to an agonist in the clinic, since withdrawal responses to tamoxifen indicate that it can become stimulatory after a perios where it inhibits growth (Howell et al. 1992). It might be expected that E would abrogate the reduction in risk of breast

10

cancer seen in women after oophorectomy. Recent data indicate that the breast tumour stem cell may have memory for reduced E since in experimental models the cells do not proliferate when returned to an oestrogenic environment (Asselin-Labat et al. 2010)

10.7 Conclusions

We have summarised the data concerning the use of E+P, E (including tibolone) in women with breast cancer and women in the general population who are (all) at risk of breast cancer. Observational studies indicate that E+P and E prevent relapse of breast cancer after surgery whereas the evidence from randomised trials indicates that HRT has no effect or stimulates relapse. For women in the general population observational studies and a large randomised trial indicate that E+P is associated with increased risk of breast cancer. In women under age of 50, including those carrying germline mutations in BRCA1/2, the limited data from observational studies indicates a reduction in risk or no significant effect. One large observational study (MWS) indicates that E (including tibolone) increases breast cancer risk whereas several observational studies and two randomised trials indicate no increased risk or a decreased risk of breast cancer. E+T is associated with an increased risk of cardiovascular disease in older women whereas several studies suggest that E+T and E are either neutral or protective in younger women. Small increases in the risks of stroke and thromb-embolism are reported at all ages. Particularly in BRCA1/2 carriers who undergo early oophorectomy, the balance of risks and benefits (including symptom relief (Madalinska et al. 2006)) appear to favour use of E until about the time of the natural menopause. The reasons for the often large differences between observational studies and randomised trials need further investigation.

References

Allen E, Doisy EA (1923) An ovarian hormone. Preliminary report on its localization, extraction and partial purification and action in test animals. JAMA 81:819–821

Anderson GL, Chlebowski RT, Rossouw JE et al (2006) Prior hormone therapy and breast cancer risk in the Women's Health Initiative randomized trail of estrogen plus progestin. Maturitas 55: 103–15

Asselin-Labat ML, Vaillant F, Sheridan JM, et al (2010) Asselin-LabatControl of mammary stem cell function by steroid hormone signalling. Nature. 2010 Apr 11. [Epub ahead of print]

Beral V, Million Study Collaborators (2003) Breast cancer and hormone-replacement therapy in the Million Women Study. Lancet 352:419–427

Bergkvist L, Adami HO, Persson I et al (1989) The risk of breast cancer after estrogen and estrogen-progestin replacement. N Engl J Med 321: 293–97

Bernstein LM, Wang P, Zheng H et al (2004) Long term exposure to tamoxifen induces sensitivity to estrdiol. Clin Cancer Res 10:1530–1534

Canfell K, Banks E, Moa AM et al (2008) Decrease in breast cancer incidence following a rapid fall in use of hormone replacement therapy in Australia. Med J Aust 188:641–644

Chen WY, Manum JE, Hankinson S et al (2006) Unopposed estrogen therapy and risk of invasive breast cancer. Arch In Med 166:1027–1032

Chlebowski RT, Hendrix SL, Langer RD et al (2003) Influence of estrogen plus progestin on breast cancer and mammography in healthy postmenopausal women: the Women's Health Initiative Randomized Trail. JAMA 289: 3243–53

Col NF, Kim JA, Chlebowski RT (2005) Menopausal hormone therapy after breast cancer: a meta-analysis and critical appraisal of the evidence. Breast Cancer Res 7:R535–R540

Collaborative Group on Hormonal Factors in Breast Cancer (1997) Breast cancer and hormone replacement therapy: collaborative reanalysis of data from 51 epidemiological studies of 52, 705 women with breast cancer and 108, 411 women without breast cancer. Lancet 350:1047–1059

Cummings SR, Ettinger B, Delmas P et al (2008) The effects of tibolone in older postmenopausal women. N Engl J Med 359:697–708

Dhodapkar MV, Ingle JN, Ahmann DL (1995) Estrogen replacement therapy withdrawal and regression of metastatic breast cancer. Cancer 75:43–46

Domchek SM, Friebel TM, Neuhausen SL et al (2006) Mortality after bilateral salpingo-oophorectomy in BRCA1 and BRCA2 mutation carriers: a prospective cohort study. Lancet Oncol 7:223–229

Dubey RK, Imthurn B, Barton M et al (2005) Vascular consequences of menopause and hormone therapy: importance of timing of treatment and type of estrogen. Cardiovasc Res 66:295–306

Eisen A, Lubinski J, Gronwald J et al (2008) Hormone therapy and the risk of breast cancer in BRCA1 mutation carriers. J Natl Cancer Inst 100:1361–1367

Ewertz M, Mellemkjaer L, Poulen AH et al (2005) Hormone use for menopausal symptoms and risk of breast cancer. A Danish cohort study. Br J Cancer 92:1293–1297

Holmberg L, Iversen OE, Rudenstam CM et al (2008) Increased risk of recurrence after hormone replacement therapy in breast cancer survivors. J Natl Cancer Inst 100:475–482

Hoover R, Gray LA Sr, Cole P et al (1976) Menopausal estrogens and breast cancer. N Engl J Med 295:401–405

Howell A, Dodwell D, Anderson H et al (1992) Response after withdrawal of tamoxifen and progestogens in advanced breast cancer. Ann Oncol 3:611–617

Kenemans P, Bundred NJ, Foidart JM et al (2009) Safety and efficacy of tibolone in breast cancer patients with vasomotor symptoms: a double-blind randomised non-inferiority trial. Lancet Oncol 10:135–146

Kurian AW, Sigal BM, Plevritis SK (2010) Survival analysis of cancer risk reduction strategies for BRCA1/2 mutation carriers. J Clin Oncol 28: 222–231

Lewis JS, Keeke K, Osipo C et al (2005) Intrinsic mechanism of estrdiol'induced osteoporosis in breast cancer cells resistant to estrogen deprivation. JNCI 97:1746–1759

Liu H, Lee ES, Gadjus C et al (2003) Apoptotic action of 17 beta-estradiol in raloxifene resistant MCF-7 cells in-vitro and in-vivo. JNCI 95:1586–1596

Lobo RA (2007) Surgical menopause and cardiovascular risks. Menopause 14:562–6

Madalinska JB, van Beurden M, Bleiker EM et al (2006) The impact of hormone replacement therapy on menopausal symptoms in younger high-risk women after prophylactic salpingo-oophorectomy. J Clin Oncol 24:3576–3582

Marsden J, Whitehead M, A'Hern R, Baum M, Sacks N (2000) Are randomizedtrials of hormone replacement therapy in symptomatic women with breast cancer feasible? Fertil Steril 73:292–299

Marshall SF, Clarke CA, Deapen D et al (2010) Recent breast cancer incidence trends according to hormone therapy use: the California Teachers Study cohort. Breast Cancer Res 12:R4

Parker WH, Broder MS, Chang E et al (2009) Ovarian conservation at the time of hysterectomy and long-term health outcomes in the nurses health study. Obstet Gynecol 113:1027–1037

Prasad R, Boland GP, Cramer A et al (2003) Short-term biologic response to withdrawal of hormone replacement therapy in patients with invasive breast cancer. Cancer 98:2539–2546

Ravdin PM, Cronin KA, Howlader N et al (2007) The decrease in breast cancer incidence in 2003 in the United States. N Engl J Med 356:1670–1674

Rebbeck TR, Friebel T, Wagner T et al (2005) Effect of short term hormone replacement therapy on breast cancer risk reduction after bilateral prophylactic oophorectomy in BRCA1 and BRCA2 mutation carriers: the PROSE Study Group. J Clin Oncol 23:7804–7810

Rivera CM, Grossardt BR, Rhodes DJ et al (2009) Increased cardiovascular mortality after bilateral oophorectomy. Menopause 16:15–23

Rossouw JE, Anderson GL, Prentice RL et al (2002) Risks and benefits of estrogen plus progestin in healthy postmenopausal women: principal results from the Women's Health Initiativerandomised controlled trial. JAMA 288:321–333

Rossouw JE, Prentice RL, Manson JE et al (2007) Postmenopausal hormone therapy and risk of cardiovascular disease by age and years since menopause. JAMA 297:1465–77

Smith DC, Prentice R, Thompson DJ et al (1975) Association of exogenous estrogen and endometrial carcinoma. N Engl J Med 293:1164–1167

Song RX, Mor G, Naftolin F et al (2001) Effect of long term oestrogen on apoptotic responses of breast cacnser cells to 17 beta-estradiol. JNCI 93:1714–1722

Stefanick ML, Anderson GL, Margolis KL et al (2006) Effects of conjugated equine estrogens on breast cancer and mammography screening in

10

postmenopausal women with hysterectomy. JAMA 295:1647–1657
The Women's Health Initiative Steering Committee (2004) The effects of conjugated euine estrogen in postmenopausal women with hysterectomy. JAMA 291:1701–1712
Von Schoultz E, Rutqvist LE, Stockholm Breast Cancer Study Group (2005) Menopausal hormone therapy after breast cancer: the Stockholm randomised trial. J Natl Cancer Inst 97:533–535

Physical Activity and Breast Cancer: Review of the Epidemiologic Evidence and Biologic Mechanisms

11

Christine M. Friedenreich

Abstract Breast cancer is the most commonly diagnosed invasive malignancy and the second leading cause of cancer death in women globally. This review considers epidemiologic evidence regarding the association between physical activity and breast cancer risk. Across these studies there was a 25% average risk reduction among physically active women as compared to the least active women. The associations were strongest for recreational activity, for activity sustained over the lifetime or done after menopause, and for activity that is of moderate to vigorous intensity and performed regularly. There is also some evidence for a stronger effect of physical activity among postmenopausal women, women who are normal weight, have no family history of breast cancer, and are parous. It is likely that physical activity is associated with decreased breast cancer risk via multiple interrelated biologic pathways that may involve adiposity, sex hormones, insulin resistance, adipokines, and chronic inflammation. Future research should include prospective observational epidemiologic studies relating proposed biomarkers to breast cancer risk and also randomized controlled trials to examine how physical activity influences the proposed biomarkers. Exercise trials will provide more clarity regarding the appropriate type, dose, and timing of activity that are related to breast cancer risk reduction.

Breast cancer remains a leading cause of cancer incidence and mortality in most developed countries worldwide. While significant international research has examined risk factors for breast cancer, most identified risk factors are nonmodifiable. During the past 20 years, over 90 studies have been conducted worldwide that have examined some aspects of the association between physical activity and breast cancer risk reduction. The purpose of this chapter is to review both the epidemiologic evidence and hypothesized biologic mechanisms whereby physical activity may influence breast cancer risk.

C.M. Friedenreich
Department of Population Health Research, Alberta Health Services-Cancer Care, 1331 29 St NW, Calgary, Alberta, T2N 4N2 Canada
and Departments of Oncology and Community Health Sciences, Faculty of Medicine, University of Calgary, Calgary, Alberta, Canada
e-mail: christine.friedenreich@albertahealthservices.ca

H.-J. Senn and F. Otto (eds.), *Clinical Cancer Prevention*,
Recent Results in Cancer Research 188, DOI: 10.1007/978-3-642-10858-7_11,

11

11.1 Epidemiologic Evidence

11.1.1 Background

Previous reviews on physical activity and breast cancer prevention have generally concluded that the evidence supporting this association is "convincing" (Friedenreich and Cust 2008; Friedenreich and Orenstein 2002; IARC Working Group 2002; Monninkhof et al. 2007a) or at least "probable" (World Cancer Research Fund and the American Institute for Cancer Research 2007). The current review paper summarizes a more detailed review just completed (Lynch et al. 2010) that incorporates 33 cohort studies and 40 case–control studies identified by February 2010 and excludes duplicate publications from the same studies.

11.1.2 Methodologic Issues in Studies of Physical Activity and Cancer

Inherent in the studies of physical activity and cancer is the difficulty in assessing usual physical activity over lifetime. A wide range of definitions of physical activity has been used in previous studies as they have not uniformly assessed all *types* of activity (i.e., occupational, household, and recreational), the *dose* of activity (frequency, intensity, and duration), or all *time periods* in life when activity was performed. Besides the difficulty in assessing physical activity, the adjustment for confounders and the assessment of effect modification by other factors or characteristics of the study population has varied considerably across these studies. Given these limitations, a formal meta-analysis of the published results cannot be undertaken since uniform exposure assessments have not been done across these observational studies.

11.1.3 Overall Associations Between Physical Activity and Breast Cancer Risk

A statistically significant breast cancer risk reduction was found in 29 of the 73 studies reviewed (40%) when comparing women who reported the highest versus lowest level of physical activity; however it was defined in these studies (Lynch et al. 2010). Eight other studies (11%) had borderline statistically significant breast cancer risk reductions and 14 (19%) observed a non-statistically significant reduction. Nineteen (26%) studies produced null effects and three (4%) studies observed a non-statistically significant increased risk of breast cancer for the most physically active women. Statistically significant risk reductions were reported more frequently in the case–control studies (16 studies from a total of 40; 40%) than in the cohort studies (14 from 35; 40%) (Figs. 11.1 and 11.2). Across all studies there was a 25% average risk reduction, with a stronger effect found in the case–control studies (an average risk reduction of 30%) than in the cohort studies (a 20% risk reduction). Of the 51 studies that found a decreased risk of breast cancer with increased levels of physical activity, 41 examined the trend of this relation and 33 of these studies found evidence for a dose–response relation between increasing levels of physical activity and decreasing breast cancer risks.

11.1.4 Type, Dose, and Timing of Activity

To formulate public health recommendations regarding the association between physical activity and breast cancer risk, a more detailed understanding from previous research is needed regarding the nature of the association by type, dose, and timing of activity. Breast cancer risk is reduced with all types of activities with the greatest reductions observed in these studies for recreational and household activity (average

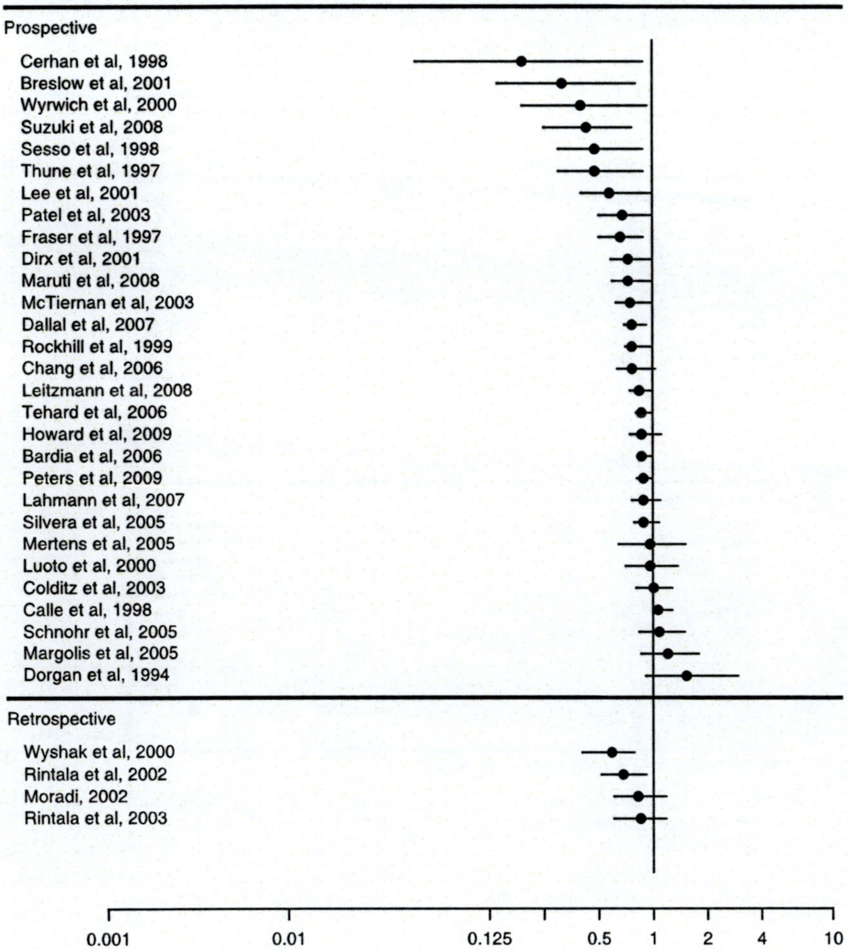

Fig. 11.1 Cohort studies of physical activity and breast cancer risk

21%) followed by walking/cycling (18%) and occupational activity (13%) (Figs. 11.3 and 11.4). Moderate intensity activity reduced risk by about 15% in these studies and vigorous-intensity activity by 18%. Increasing the duration of activity also results in a greater breast cancer risk reduction with an average 9% decreased risk found for 2–3 h/week of activity and a 30% decreased risk when six and a half hours of activity per week was achieved.

Physical activity has a beneficial effect on breast cancer risk when performed at any age throughout life, but activity done after age 50 does have a stronger effect on risk than activity done earlier in life. After age 50, average risk reductions of 17% were found in those studies that measured activity during this age period and this level of risk reduction decreased to 8% for activity done earlier in adulthood.

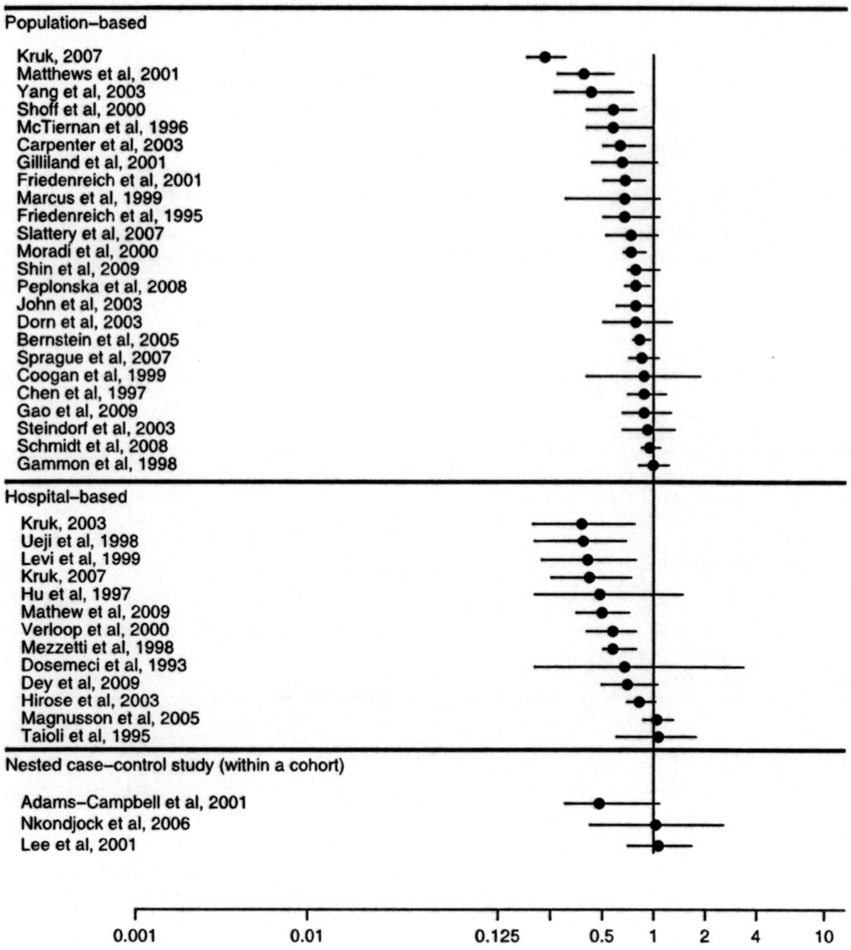

Fig. 11.2 Case–control studies of physical activity and breast cancer risk

11.1.5 Population Subgroups

Given the large number of studies that have been conducted on physical activity and breast cancer, it is also possible to consider how this association may vary across different population subgroups. This type of information may be of particular use when designing tailored public health recommendations for particular populations regarding the benefits of physical activity for their breast cancer risk reduction. Effect modification by menopausal status, body mass index (BMI; weight/height^2) race, family history of breast cancer, hormone receptor status, and parity were considered.

Breast cancer risk decreases in both pre and postmenopausal women, however, the average risk reduction is somewhat greater for postmenopausal women (31%) than among

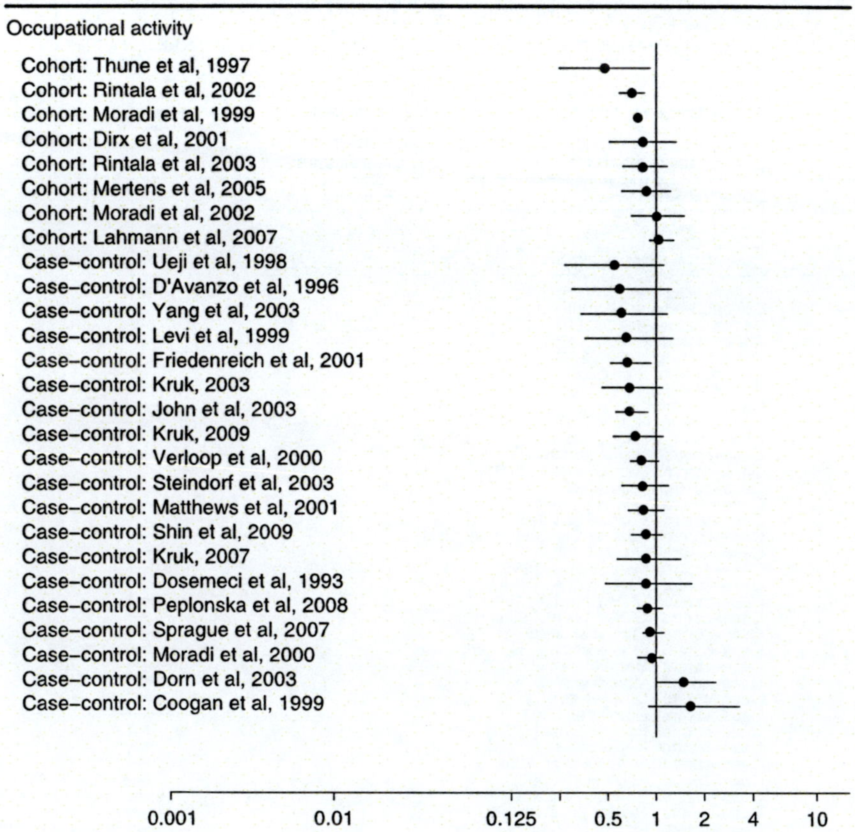

Fig. 11.3 Occupational physical activity and breast cancer risk

premenopausal women (27%). In studies that stratified their results by menopausal status, only three of 25 studies observed statistically significant decreases in breast cancer risk for both pre and postmenopausal women (Lynch et al. 2010). In 25 other studies that included either pre or postmenopausal women only, 13 studies found greater risk reductions among postmenopausal women, 11 studies found a stronger effect among premenopausal women, and one study found no difference by menopausal status (Lynch et al. 2010). It is noteworthy, however, that of these 25 studies stratified by menopausal status, 12 yielded statistically significant risk reductions in postmenopausal women, whereas only three studies showed statistically significant risk reductions in premenopausal women.

Effect modification by BMI was examined in 22 studies (Lynch et al. 2010). Physical activity had the greatest impact on breast cancer prevention among women with a lean BMI (<22) for whom the average risk reduction was 27%. For normal weight women (BMI = 22–24.9), the average risk reduction for higher physical activity levels was 24%, for overweight women (BMI = 25.0–29.9) was 18%, and for obese women (BMI > 30.0) was less than 1%.

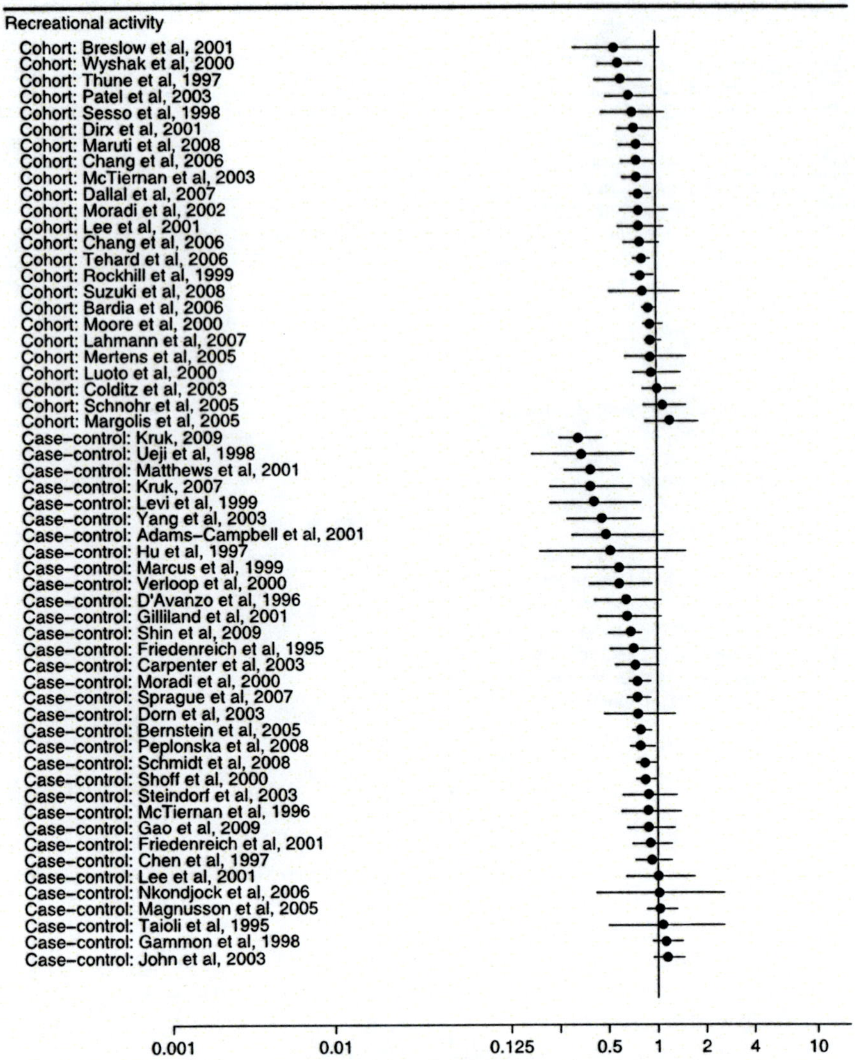

Fig. 11.4 Recreational physical activity and breast cancer risk

Physical activity exerts a beneficial effect on all racial and ethnic groups but a somewhat stronger effect has been observed in Asian women (average relative decrease of 41%) and black women (average 41%), followed by Indian women (average 38%), Hispanic women (average 28%), and white women (20%).

Only nine studies have considered whether or not family history of breast cancer influences how physical activity impacts breast cancer risk (Lynch et al. 2010). Eight of these nine studies did find evidence for effect modification by family history of breast cancer. In those studies, physical activity had a much greater benefit for women without a family history of breast cancer as compared to those with a family history since average risk reductions of 21% versus less than 1% were found, respectively, for these two groups.

Estrogen and progesterone receptor (ER, PR) status was examined in 11 studies as a potential effect modifier (Lynch et al. 2010). No clear pattern of effect modification by hormone receptor status is yet evident from these studies. More evidence for an effect of physical activity on ER+ or PR+ tumors was found than for ER- or PR-tumors when these receptors are examined separately. However, when the combined hormone receptor status was considered, statistically significant risk reductions were found in only one ER+/PR+ study and one ER-/PR- study. Average risk reductions were greater for women with ER-/PR- tumors (27%) than for women with ER+/PR+ tumors (14%).

Effect modification by parity was examined in only seven studies with a greater risk reduction found among physically active parous women (average decrease in breast cancer risk 38%) than nulliparous women (average decrease 18%).

11.1.6 Summary of Epidemiologic Findings

A review of the epidemiologic findings for physical activity and breast cancer is limited by the heterogeneous activity assessment methods used, the variable study quality, and reporting of study results which compromises the ability to make direct comparisons across studies. This narrative review was restricted to using crude averages of risk reductions as a means of evaluating the magnitude of the effect of physical activity on breast cancer risk.

With these limitations in mind, a conservative estimate of the effect of physical activity and breast cancer risk is a 25% decrease in risk for physically active women. When examining the effect by type, dose, and timing of activity, the greatest reductions are found for recreational and household activities, for activities of longer duration, of at least moderate intensity, and for activity done after menopause. However, risk reductions were apparent for all types of activity, for lower doses of activity and for activity undertaken across the entire lifespan. The effect of physical activity on breast cancer risk is also somewhat stronger for postmenopausal women, for all body sizes with the exception of obese women, for women of non-Caucasian backgrounds, for women without a family history of breast cancer and for parous women. There was no clear effect modification of the association between physical activity and breast cancer risk by hormone receptor status.

Given the consistency, strength, and evidence for dose–response that has been observed in these epidemiologic studies, an argument has been made that randomized controlled exercise intervention trials (RCTs) are now needed to advance understanding of how physical activity influences breast cancer (Friedenreich 2001). Three intervention trials have been conducted to date in postmenopausal women who are free of breast cancer to examine how aerobic exercise affects the biologic mechanisms that are hypothesized to be part of the pathway between physical activity and breast cancer risk (Friedenreich et al. 2010a; McTiernan et al. 1999; Monninkhof et al. 2007b). These two-armed trials have each compared a supervised, aerobic exercise intervention to no activity in postmenopausal women. Body composition, metabolic and sex steroid hormones, growth factors, inflammation and insulin resistance biomarkers, and mammographic density were measured in each group to determine the impact of exercise on these biomarkers. These RCTs, known as the Physical Activity for Total Health (PATH) trial ($n = 173$) (McTiernan et al. 1999), the Sex Hormones and Physical Exercise (SHAPE) trial ($n = 189$) (Monninkhof et al. 2007b), and the Alberta Physical Activity and Breast Cancer Prevention (ALPHA) trial ($n = 320$) (Friedenreich et al. 2010a), administered moderate- to vigorous-intensity physical activity interventions ranging from 150 to 225 min/week over

12 months. These studies have provided direct evidence on the effects of exercise on these biomarkers, with more published results anticipated in the future. The findings published to date are described in the relevant sections below in the full description of the hypothesized biologic mechanisms operating between physical activity and breast cancer risk.

11.2 Biologic Mechanisms

Several hypothesized biologic pathways relating physical activity to breast cancer risk have been proposed (McTiernan 2008; Neilson et al. 2009; Rogers et al. 2008; Thompson et al. 2009; Wetmore and Ulrich 2006), but definitive evidence regarding these pathways has been emerging only recently. Given the multifactorial etiology of breast cancer, it is likely that many interrelated pathways are involved in reducing breast cancer risk. It is also possible that certain mechanisms predominate with specific doses or types of physical activity or perhaps in select subgroups of women, as presented earlier in this review. The primary hypotheses involve an impact of physical activity on adiposity, sex hormones, insulin resistance, adipokines, and inflammatory markers.

11.2.1 Adiposity

The role of adiposity as a mediator of the effect of physical activity on breast cancer risk is a central component of these hypothesized pathways because of the well-established association between weight, body fat levels, and weight gain and postmenopausal breast cancer risk (Renehan et al. 2008; World Cancer Research Fund and the American Institute for Cancer Research 2007). Physical activity may influence breast cancer risk through weight loss in overweight women or in weight maintenance in normal weight women (Donnelly et al. 2009; Lau et al. 2007) and there is emerging evidence that physical activity may achieve abdominal fat loss with the right exercise prescription (e.g., (Cuff et al. 2003; Giannopoulou et al. 2005; Irwin et al. 2003)). The PATH and ALPHA trials demonstrated a clear exercise effect in a range of body composition measures (Friedenreich et al. 2010b; Irwin et al. 2003) including abdominal fat, whereas the SHAPE trial found that exercisers decreased body fat and waist circumference, but not weight, in comparison to controls (Velthuis et al. 2009). Therefore, fat loss is a logical explanation for the association between exercise and postmenopausal breast cancer risk.

One currently hypothesized biologic model for postmenopausal breast cancer risk, focusing mainly on the promotion and progression of initiated cells, implicates sex hormones, insulin resistance, adipokines, and chronic inflammation as possible mediators of physical activity (Neilson et al. 2009) (Fig. 11.5). While all of the proposed biomarkers in this model are associated with adiposity, and specifically abdominal fat, many of them are also influenced by exercise irrespective of body fat changes. Hence, the extent to which fat loss is necessary to derive a significant risk benefit from exercise remains a matter of controversy.

11.2.2 Sex Hormones

The role of endogenous estrogens in breast cancer etiology is well recognized since estrogens inhibit apoptosis, act as mitogens in the breast (Lorincz and Sukumar 2006; Yager and Davidson 2006), and antiestrogenic drugs are successfully used to treat women with ER+ breast tumors (Uray and Brown 2006). In addition, there is compelling evidence from observational studies for a positive association between breast cancer risk and estrogens in postmenopausal women. Estradiol and estrone have been clearly shown to

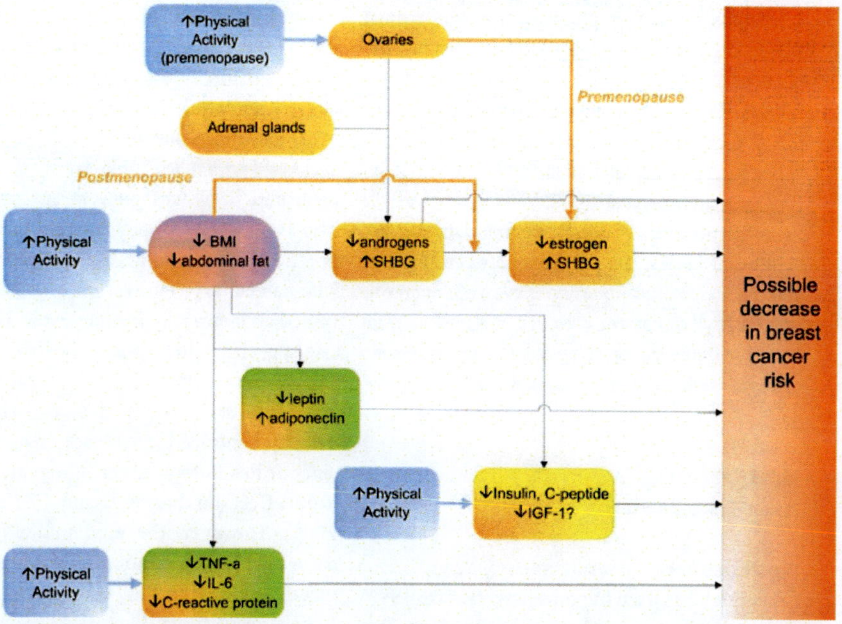

Fig. 11.5 Hypothesized biologic model relating proposed biomarkers of risk to long-term exercise in pre and postmenopausal women (adapted from Neilson et al. 2009)

double postmenopausal breast cancer risk (Key et al. 2002). Physical activity may impact on endogenous estrogen levels through several mechanisms: by reducing body fat levels (the main source of estrogen production after menopause); altering adipokine levels that influence estrogen production (Cleary and Grossmann 2009); and lowering blood insulin levels thereby increasing circulating sex hormone binding globulin (SHBG) (Kaaks 1996; Pugeat et al. 1991), which binds reversibly to estrogens to affect their bioavailability. In premenopausal women, it is hypothesized that physical activity may delay menarche, decrease ovulation, and increase amenorrhea, which would result in a lower lifetime exposure to endogenous estrogens and lowering of breast cancer risk (Bernstein 2009; Campbell and McTiernan 2007).

Breast cancer risk may also be affected by endogenous androgen levels since androgens can have a direct effect on breast cell growth (Nicolas Diaz-Chico et al. 2007) and an indirect effect via estrogen production since androgens can be converted to estrogens (Kendall et al. 2007). Observational studies have found an independent effect of testosterone on breast cancer risk even after adjustment for estradiol levels with a doubling in risk of breast cancer for women at the highest serum androgen levels (Kaaks et al. 2005; Key et al. 2002). As with estrogens, physical activity may lower testosterone levels by decreasing adiposity or by increasing SHBG levels via lowered blood insulin levels

Some evidence now exists from two RCTs that the effect of physical activity on sex hormones varies by changes in body fat. In the PATH and SHAPE trials, women randomized to the exercise group who lost more than 2% body fat experienced significantly lower blood estrogen levels compared with controls after 12 and 4 months of exercise, respectively (McTiernan et al. 2004a; McTiernan et al. 2004b; Monninkhof et al. 2009). In the ALPHA trial, estrogen levels decreased significantly more in exercisers than in controls after

12 months, even after adjusting for weight change suggesting a role for physical activity that is independent of adiposity changes (Friedenreich et al. 2010a). Similarly, some cross-sectional studies (Cauley et al. 1989; Chan et al. 2007; Madigan et al. 1998; Verkasalo et al. 2001), but not all (Bertone-Johnson et al. 2009; Van Gils et al. 2009) in postmenopausal women have found statistically significant inverse associations between physical activity and sex hormone levels even after controlling for BMI or adiposity. Hence, it is unclear if fat loss is a required prerequisite for sex hormone changes induced by physical activity.

11.2.3 Insulin-Related Factors

A pathway between insulin resistance and breast cancer risk has been hypothesized (Kaaks 1996) and several lines of evidence support this hypothesis. To begin, insulin has mitotic and antiapototic effects in breast cancer cells (Lann and LeRoith 2008; Osborne et al. 1976). Second, hyperinsulinemia decreases SHBG levels, which thereby increases the bioavailability of sex hormones (Kaaks 1996; Pugeat et al. 1991). Third, insulin resistance and hyperinsulinemia are also strongly related to obesity (Haslam and James 2005) and specifically intra-abdominal fat (Kaaks 1996) as well as various adipokines and inflammatory factors (Rose et al. 2004; Vona-Davis et al. 2007), which have all been associated with breast cancer risk. Hence, insulin may alter breast cancer risk independently or indirectly through other biomarkers of risk.

The epidemiologic evidence regarding the role of insulin in breast cancer risk is growing but remains inconclusive with some evidence for an increased breast cancer risk in women with type 2 diabetes (Larsson et al. 2007; Xue and Michels 2007) and inconsistent evidence for the association between breast cancer risk and insulin or C-peptide (Gunter et al. 2009; Kabat et al. 2009; Neilson et al. 2009; Pisani 2008; Xue and Michels 2007).

Exercise combined with weight loss is generally accepted as an effective means for improving insulin sensitivity and preventing diabetes (Ivy 1997; Klein et al. 2004; Ryan 2000; Warburton et al. 2007). In the PATH trial, insulin levels decreased with moderate exercise and the change in insulin level was greatest among exercisers who also lost >2 kg body fat over the year (Frank et al. 2005). In addition, among those women who gained body fat over the year, exercise prevented an increase in insulin levels. Hence, exercise appears to alter insulin levels through weight change and also independently of fat loss.

Insulin-like growth factor-1 (IGF-1) has been hypothesized to increase breast cancer risk since it has both a direct mitogenic and apoptotic effect on breast tissue (Yu and Rohan 2000). However, the epidemiologic evidence for a positive association with breast cancer is inconsistent (Eliassen and Hankinson 2008; Fletcher et al. 2005; Lann and LeRoith 2008) as is the association with physical activity on IGF-1 and IGF-binding protein-3 (IGFBP-3) (McTiernan et al. 2005; Orenstein and Friedenreich 2004; Tworoger et al. 2007b). Thus, the IGFs may not be important biologic mechanisms mediating the impact of physical activity on breast cancer risk.

11.2.4 Adipokines and Inflammation

Adipokines, specifically leptin, adiponectin, tumor necrosis factor-alpha (TNF-α), and interleukin-6 (IL-6) are polypeptides produced by adipocytes that may increase breast cancer risk through direct mechanisms, through associations with insulin resistance or in some cases, by enhancing estrogen activity (Neilson et al. 2009). Inflammatory markers, including TNF-α and IL-6 and C-reactive protein (CRP), are all elevated with obesity, which is a chronic low-grade, systemic inflammatory state (Lee and Pratley 2005). Chronic inflammation is hypothesized to increase cancer risk by deregulating normal cell growth that can promote initiated cells to malignancy through its impact on increased cell proliferation, microenvironmental changes and oxidative stress (Coussens and Werb 2002).

Although biological plausibility exists for an etiologic role of adipokines in breast carcinogenesis, there is currently little epidemiologic evidence for an association between breast cancer risk and adipokines and inflammatory markers (Neilson et al. 2009). The evidence is somewhat stronger for adiponectin than for leptin but for both adipokines, the evidence remains limited (Barb et al. 2007; Cust et al. 2009; Stattin et al. 2004; Tworoger et al. 2007a).

Exercise trials conducted with various study populations have generally found no effect of exercise on inflammatory markers, however, conclusions regarding these associations are difficult to make because of the differing study designs and study populations (Wetmore and Ulrich 2006). The PATH trial found that a 12-month exercise intervention lowered leptin (Frank et al. 2005) and CRP (Campbell et al. 2009) levels, but CRP was decreased only among obese women or those with abdominal obesity who lost body fat. Other exercise RCTs have, however, achieved decreases in adipokine and CRP levels independent of fat loss (Balducci et al. 2009; You et al. 2004). Hence, it remains unclear if changes in adipokine and inflammatory markers are dependent on changes in body fat.

11.2.5 Other Mechanisms

Several other biologic mechanisms that cause DNA damage, cancer initiation, promotion, or progression have been hypothesized to explain how physical activity influences breast cancer risk (Rundle 2005). For some pathways, such as mammographic density, that have been strongly associated with breast cancer risk, there is no convincing evidence that exercise impacts these mechanisms (Atkinson et al. 2004; Campbell et al. 2007; Schmitz et al. 2008; Woolcott et al. 2010). Physical activity may impact breast cancer risk by decreasing oxidative stress (Dai et al. 2009; Schmitz et al. 2008), enhancing immune function (Campbell et al. 2008; Wetmore and Ulrich 2006), reducing promoter hypermethylation of tumor suppressor genes or by reducing genotoxicity from estrogen metabolite-DNA adducts formed in breast tissue (Coyle 2008). Exercise may also have a favorable effect on some intracellular signaling pathways by suppressing procarcinogenic pathways and promoting anticarcinogenic pathways (Thompson et al. 2009). Finally, genetic factors may also modify the effect of exercise on these biomarkers and may be important to consider when examining their etiologic role in the association between physical activity and breast cancer.

11.3 Conclusion

There is now strong and consistent evidence from 73 studies conducted worldwide that physical activity reduces breast cancer risk by about 25% and that a dose–response effect exists. Several plausible biologic mechanisms are emerging involving adiposity, sex and metabolic hormones, insulin, inflammation, and adipokines to explain this association. The evidence from randomized exercise intervention trials that have examined these biomarkers is particularly useful in understanding these associations. While all types of activities and different doses of activity appear to reduce breast cancer risk, somewhat stronger risk reductions are evident with recreational activity, activity that is at least of moderate intensity and performed regularly and that is sustained over lifetime or at least after menopause. Some evidence also exists now that physical activity may have a stronger effect in postmenopausal women, normal weight women, non-Caucasians, parous women, and women without a family history of breast cancer.

11

Future research in this field should examine how sedentary behavior and light-intensity activity are related to breast cancer risk. Improvements in quantifying physical activity with objective measurements as well as more precision regarding the type, dose, and timing of activity over lifetime is also needed for a better understanding of the nature of these associations. Future investigations of the effect modification of this association by other factors will clarify some of the complexity of these associations. There is also a need for prospective observational epidemiologic studies relating new and proposed biomarkers to breast cancer risk and additional randomized controlled exercise intervention trials that evaluate biomarker changes with different types and doses of physical activities to elucidate further how activity influences breast cancer risk. The ultimate objective of this research is to provide more quantitative data that can be used to enhance the public health recommendations regarding the type, dose, and timing of physical activity required to reduce breast cancer risk.

Acknowledgments Dr. Christine Friedenreich is supported by a Health Senior Scholar Award from the Alberta Heritage Foundation for Medical Research. The author wishes to thank Dr. Brigid Lynch and Heather Neilson for their assistance in the writing of this review and Qinggang Wang for the preparation of the figures.

References

Atkinson C, Lampe JW, Tworoger SS et al (2004) Effects of a moderate intensity exercise intervention on estrogen metabolism in postmenopausal women. Cancer Epidemiol Biomark Prev 13:868–874

Balducci S, Zanuso S, Nicolucci A et al (2009) Anti-inflammatory effect of exercise training in subjects with type 2 diabetes and the metabolic syndrome is dependent on exercise modalities and independent of weight loss. Nutr Metab Cardiovasc Dis doi:10.1016/j.numecd.2009.04.015

Barb D, Williams CJ, Neuwirth AK et al (2007) Adiponectin in relation to malignancies: a review of existing basic research and clinical evidence. Am J Clin Nutr 86:s858–s866

Bernstein L (2009) Exercise and breast cancer prevention. Curr Oncol Rep 11:490–496

Bertone-Johnson ER, Tworoger SS, Hankinson SE (2009) Recreational physical activity and steroid hormone levels in postmenopausal women. Am J Epidemiol 170:1095–1104

Campbell KL, McTiernan A (2007) Exercise and biomarkers for cancer prevention studies. J Nutr 137:161S–169S

Campbell KL, Westerlind KC, Harber VJ et al (2007) Effects of aerobic exercise training on estrogen metabolism in premenopausal women: a randomized controlled trial. Cancer Epidemiol Biomark Prev 16:731–739

Campbell PT, Wener MH, Sorensen B et al (2008) Effect of exercise on in vitro immune function: a 12-month randomized, controlled trial among postmenopausal women. J Appl Physiol 104: 1648–1655

Campbell PT, Campbell KL, Wener MH et al (2009) A yearlong exercise intervention decreases CRP among obese postmenopausal women. Med Sci Sports Exerc 41:1533–1539

Cauley JA, Gutai JP, Kuller LH et al (1989) The epidemiology of serum sex hormones in postmenopausal women. Am J Epidemiol 129:1120–1131

Chan MF, Dowsett M, Folkerd E et al (2007) Usual physical activity and endogenous sex hormones in postmenopausal women: the European Prospective Investigation into Cancer-Norfolk population study. Cancer Epidemiol Biomark Prev 16:900–905

Cleary MP, Grossmann ME (2009) Minireview: obesity and breast cancer: the estrogen connection. Endocrinology 150:2537–2542

Coussens LM, Werb Z (2002) Inflammation and cancer. Nature 420:860–867

Coyle YM (2008) Physical activity as a negative modulator of estrogen-induced breast cancer. Cancer Causes Control 19:1021–1029

Cuff DJ, Meneilly GS, Martin A et al (2003) Effective exercise modality to reduce insulin resistance in women with type 2 diabetes. Diab Care 26:2977–2982

Cust AE, Stocks T, Lukanova A et al (2009) The influence of overweight and insulin resistance on breast cancer risk and tumour stage at diagnosis: a prospective study. Breast Cancer Res Treat 113:567–576

Dai Q, Gao YT, Shu XO et al (2009) Oxidative stress, obesity, and breast cancer risk: results from the Shanghai Women's Health Study. J Clin Oncol 27:2482–2488

Donnelly JE, Blair SN, Jakicic JM et al (2009) American College of Sports Medicine Position Stand. Appropriate physical activity intervention strategies for weight loss and prevention of weight regain for adults. Med Sci Sports Exerc 41:459–471

Eliassen AH, Hankinson SE (2008) Endogenous hormone levels and risk of breast, endometrial and ovarian cancers: prospective studies. Adv Exp Med Biol 630:148–165

Fletcher O, Gibson L, Johnson N et al (2005) Polymorphisms and circulating levels in the insulin-like growth factor system and risk of breast cancer: a systematic review. Cancer Epidemiol Biomark Prev 14:2–19

Frank LL, Sorensen BE, Yasui Y et al (2005) Effects of exercise on metabolic risk variables in overweight postmenopausal women: a randomized clinical trial. Obes Res 13:615–625

Friedenreich CM (2001) Physical activity and cancer prevention: from observational to intervention research. Cancer Epidemiol Biomark Prev 10:287–301

Friedenreich CM, Cust AE (2008) Physical activity and breast cancer risk: impact of timing, type and dose of activity and population subgroup effects. Brit J Sports Med 42:636–647

Friedenreich CM, Orenstein MR (2002) Physical activity and cancer prevention: etiologic evidence and biological mechanisms. J Nutr 132:3456S–3464S

Friedenreich CM, Woolcott CG, McTiernan A (2010a). Alberta physical activity and breast cancer prevention trial: sex hormone changes in a year-long exercise intervention among postmenopausal women. J Clin Oncol. 28:1458–66

Friedenreich CM, Woolcott CG, McTiernan A et al (2010b) Adiposity changes after a one year aerobic exercise intervention among postmenopausal women: randomized controlled trial. Int J Obes (in press)

Giannopoulou I, Ploutz-Snyder LL, Carhart R et al (2005) Exercise is required for visceral fat loss in postmenopausal women with type 2 diabetes. J Clin Endocrinol Metab 90:1511–1518

Gunter MJ, Hoover DR, Yu H et al (2009) Insulin, insulin-like growth factor-I, and risk of breast cancer in postmenopausal women. J Natl Cancer Inst 101:48–60

Haslam DW, James WP (2005) Obesity. Lancet 366:1197–1209

IARC Working Group (2002) IARC handbook of cancer prevention, volume 6: weight control and physical activity. IARC, Lyon

Irwin ML, Yasui Y, Ulrich CM et al (2003) Effect of exercise on total and intra-abdominal body fat in postmenopausal women: a randomized controlled trial. JAMA 289:323–330

Ivy JL (1997) Role of exercise training in the prevention and treatment of insulin resistance and non-insulin-dependent diabetes mellitus. Sports Med 24:321–336

Kaaks R (1996) Nutrition, hormones, and breast cancer: is insulin the missing link? Cancer Causes Control 7:605–625

Kaaks R, Rinaldi S, Key TJ et al (2005) Postmenopausal serum androgens, oestrogens and breast cancer risk: the European prospective investigation into cancer and nutrition. Endocr Relat Cancer 12:1071–1082

Kabat GC, Kim M, Caan BJ et al (2009) Repeated measures of serum glucose and insulin in relation to postmenopausal breast cancer. Int J Cancer 125:2704–2710

Kendall A, Folkerd EJ, Dowsett M (2007) Influences on circulating oestrogens in postmenopausal women: relationship with breast cancer. J Steroid Biochem Mol Biol 103:99–109

Key T, Appleby P, Barnes I et al (2002) Endogenous sex hormones and breast cancer in postmenopausal women: reanalysis of nine prospective studies. J Natl Cancer Inst 94:606–616

Klein S, Sheard NF, Pi-Sunyer X et al (2004) Weight management through lifestyle modification for the prevention and management of type 2 diabetes: rationale and strategies: a statement of the American Diabetes Association, the North American Association for the Study of Obesity, and the American Society for Clinical Nutrition. Diab Care 27:2067–2073

Lann D, LeRoith D (2008) The role of endocrine insulin-like growth factor-I and insulin in breast cancer. J Mammary Gland Biol Neoplasia 13:371–379

Larsson SC, Mantzoros CS, Wolk A (2007) Diabetes mellitus and risk of breast cancer: a meta-analysis. Int J Cancer 121:856–862

Lau DC, Douketis JD, Morrison KM et al (2007) 2006 Canadian clinical practice guidelines on the management and prevention of obesity in adults and children [summary]. CMAJ 176: S1–S13

Lee YH, Pratley RE (2005) The evolving role of inflammation in obesity and the metabolic syndrome. Curr Diab Rep 5:70–75

Lorincz AM, Sukumar S (2006) Molecular links between obesity and breast cancer. Endocr Relat Cancer 13:279–292

Lynch BM, Nielson HK, Friedenreich, CM (2010). Chapter 2: Physical Activity and Breast Cancer Prevention. In Courneya KS, Friedenreich CM (Eds). *Volume 184: Physical Activity and Cancer. Recent Results in Cancer Research*. Springer-Verlag Berlin Heidelberg (in press).

Madigan MP, Troisi R, Potischman N et al (1998) Serum hormone levels in relation to reproductive and lifestyle factors in postmenopausal women (United States). Cancer Causes Control 9:199–207

McTiernan A (2008) Mechanisms linking physical activity with cancer. Nat Rev Cancer 8:205–211

McTiernan A, Ulrich CM, Yancey D et al (1999) The Physical Activity for Total Health (PATH) Study: rationale and design. Med Sci Sports Exerc 31:1307–1312

McTiernan A, Tworoger SS, Rajan KB et al (2004a) Effect of exercise on serum androgens in postmenopausal women: a 12-month randomized clinical trial. Cancer Epidemiol Biomark Prev 13:1099–1105

McTiernan A, Tworoger SS, Ulrich CM et al (2004b) Effect of exercise on serum estrogens in postmenopausal women: a 12-month randomized clinical trial. Cancer Res 64:2923–2928

McTiernan A, Sorensen B, Yasui Y et al (2005) No effect of exercise on insulin-like growth factor 1 and insulin-like growth factor binding protein 3 in postmenopausal women: a 12-month randomized clinical trial. Cancer Epidemiol Biomark Prev 14:1020–1021

Monninkhof EM, Elias SG, Vlems FA et al (2007a) Physical activity and breast cancer: a systematic review. Epidemiology 18:137–157

Monninkhof EM, Peeters PH, Schuit AJ (2007b) Design of the sex hormones and physical exercise (SHAPE) study. BMC Public Health 7

Monninkhof EM, Velthuis MJ, Peeters PH et al (2009) Effect of exercise on postmenopausal sex hormone levels and role of body fat: a randomized controlled trial. J Clin Oncol 27: 4492–4499

Neilson HK, Friedenreich CM, Brockton NT et al (2009) Physical activity and postmenopausal breast cancer: proposed biologic mechanisms and areas for future research. Cancer Epidemiol Biomark Prev 18:11–27

Nicolas Diaz-Chico B, German RF, Gonzalez A et al (2007) Androgens and androgen receptors in breast cancer. J Steroid Biochem Mol Biol 105:1–15

Orenstein MR, Friedenreich CM (2004) Review of physical activity and the IGF family. J Phys Act Health 1:291–320

Osborne CK, Bolan G, Monaco ME et al (1976) Hormone responsive human breast cancer in long-term tissue culture: effect of insulin. Proc Natl Acad Sci USA 73:4536–4540

Pisani P (2008) Hyper-insulinaemia and cancer, meta-analyses of epidemiological studies. Arch Physiol Biochem 114:63–70

Pugeat M, Crave JC, Elmidani M et al (1991) Pathophysiology of sex hormone binding globulin (SHBG): relation to insulin. J Steroid Biochem Mol Biol 40:841–849

Renehan AG, Tyson M, Egger M et al (2008) Body-mass index and incidence of cancer: a systematic review and meta-analysis of prospective observational studies. Lancet 371:569–578

Rogers CJ, Colbert LH, Greiner JW et al (2008) Physical activity and cancer prevention: pathways and targets for intervention. Sports Med 38:271–296

Rose DP, Komninou D, Stephenson GD (2004) Obesity, adipocytokines, and insulin resistance in breast cancer. Obes Rev 5:153–165

Rundle A (2005) Molecular epidemiology of physical activity and cancer. Cancer Epidemiol Biomark Prev 14:227–236

Ryan AS (2000) Insulin resistance with aging: effects of diet and exercise. Sports Med 30:327–346

Schmitz KH, Warren M, Rundle AG et al (2008) Exercise effect on oxidative stress is independent of change in estrogen metabolism. Cancer Epidemiol Biomark Prev 17:220–223

Stattin P, Soderberg S, Biessy C et al (2004) Plasma leptin and breast cancer risk: a prospective study in northern Sweden. Breast Cancer Res Treat 86:191–196

Thompson HJ, Jiang W, Zhu Z (2009) Candidate mechanisms accounting for effects of physical activity on breast carcinogenesis. IUBMB Life 61:895–901

Tworoger SS, Eliassen AH, Kelesidis T et al (2007a) Plasma adiponectin concentrations and risk of incident breast cancer. J Clin Endocrinol Metab 92:1510–1516

Tworoger SS, Missmer SA, Eliassen AH et al (2007b) Physical activity and inactivity in relation to sex hormone, prolactin, and insulin-like growth factor concentrations in premenopausal women – exercise and premenopausal hormones. Cancer Causes Control 18:743–752

Uray IP, Brown PH (2006) Prevention of breast cancer: current state of the science and future opportunities. Expert Opin Investig Drugs 15: 1583–1600

Van Gils CH, Peeters PH, Schoenmakers MC et al (2009) Physical activity and endogenous sex hormone levels in postmenopausal women: a cross-sectional study in the Prospect-EPIC Cohort. Cancer Epidemiol Biomark Prev 18:377–383

Velthuis MJ, Schuit AJ, Peeters PH et al (2009) Exercise program affects body composition but not weight in postmenopausal women. Menopause 16:777–784

Verkasalo PK, Thomas HV, Appleby PN et al (2001) Circulating levels of sex hormones and their relation to risk factors for breast cancer: a cross-sectional study in 1092 pre- and postmenopausal women (United Kingdom). Cancer Causes Control 12:47–59

Vona-Davis L, Howard-McNatt M, Rose DP (2007) Adiposity, type 2 diabetes and the metabolic syndrome in breast cancer. Obes Rev 8:395–408

Warburton DE, Katzmarzyk PT, Rhodes RE et al (2007) Evidence-informed physical activity guidelines for Canadian adults. Can J Public Health 98(Suppl 2):S16–S68

Wetmore CM, Ulrich CM (2006) Mechanisms associating physical activity with cancer incidence: exercise and immune function. In: McTiernan A (ed) Cancer prevention and management through exercise and weight control. CRC Press/Taylor & Francis, Boca Raton

Woolcott CG, Courneya KS, Boyd NF et al (2010) Mammographic density change with 1 year of aerobic exercise among postmenopausal women: a randomized controlled trial. Cancer Epidemiol Biomarkers Prev 19:1112–21

World Cancer Research Fund and the American Institute for Cancer Research (2007) Food, nutrition, physical activity, and the prevention of cancer: a global perspective. American Institute for Cancer Research, Washington, DC

Xue F, Michels KB (2007) Diabetes, metabolic syndrome, and breast cancer: a review of the current evidence. Am J Clin Nutr 86:s823–s835

Yager JD, Davidson NE (2006) Estrogen carcinogenesis in breast cancer. N Engl J Med 354:270–282

You T, Berman DM, Ryan AS et al (2004) Effects of hypocaloric diet and exercise training on inflammation and adipocyte lipolysis in obese postmenopausal women. J Clin Endocrinol Metab 89:1739–1746

Yu H, Rohan T (2000) Role of the insulin-like growth factor family in cancer development and progression. J Natl Cancer Inst 92: 1472–1489

Prevention of Breast Cancer by Newer SERMs in the Future

12

Trevor Powles

Abstract The selective oestrogen receptor modulators (SERMs) tamoxifen has been shown to reduce the incidence of oestrogen receptor positive breast cancer by about 60 to 70% in healthy high risk women. The oestrogenic effects of tamoxifen caused a beneficial effect of reduced bone loss and fracture risk in postmenopausal women. However there was also significant gynaecological toxicity including an increased risk of endometrial cancer. Further clinical trials have evaluated the newer SERMs raloxifene, arzoxifene and lasofoxifene. The latter has been shown to significantly reduce the incidence of breast cancer, vertebral and non vertebral fractures, major coronary events and stroke with no significant gynaecological toxicity.

12.1 Introduction

Clinical trials using selective estrogen receptor modulators (SERMs) in healthy women to prevent breast cancer started in 1986 and have now involved more than 90,000 women. Tamoxifen, a SERM, has predominantly anti-oestrogenic activity on breast cancer and when used in breast cancer prevention trials in healthy women reduces the incidence of invasive ER-positive breast cancer by about 60%. There was no reduction in the incidence of ER-negative cancers. Tamoxifen, predominantly has oestrogenic activity on other tissues in the body causing a reduction in cholesterol and bone loss together with an increased risk of venous thromboembolism (VTE) and endometrial cancer. There is no apparent beneficial effect on coronary heart disease (CHD) (Fisher et al. 1998; Cuzick et al. 2002).

The second-generation SERM raloxifene, developed as a treatment for osteoporosis, has similar preclinical activity to tamoxifen and has been shown to reduce vertebral fracture risk and breast cancer risk but with no increase in endometrial cancer (Cummings et al. 1998; Vogel et al. 2006). As a result of these trials tamoxifen has been approved by the Food and Drugs Agency in the USA for risk reduction of breast cancer in women with a Gail score risk of breast cancer >1.65% at 5 years. Raloxifene has been approved by the Food and Drugs Agency in the USA for fracture risk reduction in osteoporotic women and breast cancer risk reduction in postmenopausal women. The European Medicines Agency has approved raloxifene for fracture risk reduction. However

T. Powles
Parkside Oncology Clinic, London, UK
e-mail: hilary.dummer@parkside-hospital.co.uk

H.-J. Senn and F. Otto (eds.), *Clinical Cancer Prevention*,
Recent Results in Cancer Research 188, DOI: 10.1007/978-3-642-10858-7_12,

these drugs have not been widely used to prevent breast cancer. This is in part because, although the side effects are minimal, very large number of women need to take the medication in order to prevent a relatively small number of breast cancers and in part because the benefits on fracture risk reduction is modest. Because of these doubts, further clinical studies have been undertaken with two newer SERMs, arzoxifene and lasofoxifene, with possibly more potent beneficial effects and/or wider spectrum of benefits with potentially less toxicity in well women.

12.2 Arzoxifene

Preclinical and early clinical data indicate that arzoxifene, a third-generation SERM, is more potent and bioavailable than raloxifene and is clinically active as a treatment for advanced breast cancer (Sato et al. 1998; Suh et al. 2001; Baselga et al. 2003; Buzdar et al. 2003; Fabian et al. 2004; Deshmane et al. 2007). The GENERATIONS trial was therefore undertaken to evaluate arzoxifene for prevention of osteoporotic fractures and breast cancer. The design was a phase 3, multicenter, placebo-controlled, double-blind trial and the results were reported at San Antonio in 2009 (Powles et al. 2009). The 9354 participants were postmenopausal women with osteoporosis (N = 5252) or low bone mineral density (BMD) (N = 4102) randomly assigned to arzoxifene 20 mg/day (N = 4676) or placebo (N = 4678). The primary outcomes were radiographic vertebral fracture in the osteoporotic population and invasive breast cancer in all study participants. After all participants had completed 48 months of treatment there was a reported 41% reduction in the incidence of vertebral fractures ($p < 0.001$) and 56% percent reduction in incidence of invasive breast cancer ($p = 0.002$). The breast cancer risk reduction with arzoxifene was similar between Gail risk groups and between low bone mass and osteoporosis groups. The risk reduction was seen only for invasive ER-positive breast cancers with a nil effect for ER-negative breast cancers. Other findings included no significant reduction in nonvertebral fractures or cardiovascular events. Generally, arzoxifene was well tolerated, although there was a significant increase in venous thromboembolism, gall bladder disease, pulmonary obstructive/infective disorders, hot flushes, muscle cramps, and gynecologic-related events in the arzoxifene group. In summary arzoxifene treatment for 4 years significantly reduced the incidence of invasive breast cancer by 56% and ER-positive invasive breast cancer by 70% in osteoporotic/osteopenic, postmenopausal women. There was also a significant reduction in the incidence of vertebral fractures in postmenopausal women with osteoporosis but no significant reduction in the incidence of nonvertebral fractures, cardiovascular events including coronary events or stroke and an increased incidence of venous-thromboembolic events, gynecologic-related events, hot flushes, and leg cramps. It was concluded that the overall benefit/risk profile of arzoxifene did not represent a meaningful advancement in the treatment of osteoporosis but the trial did provide further support for a significant risk reduction of invasive ER-positive breast cancer by SERMs in postmenopausal women.

12.3 Lasofoxifene

Lasofoxifene is another more potent third-generation SERM, which in preclinical studies reduced bone loss and serum cholesterol and prevented breast cancer with no uterine hypertrophy.

Early clinical studies with lasofoxifene indicated that it was more potent than raloxifene in reducing bone loss and serum cholesterol with no increase in endometrial cancer risk (Ke et al. 2004; McClung et al. 2006). The PEARL trial was therefore set up to evaluate arzoxifene for prevention of osteoporotic fractures and breast cancer. The design was a phase 3, multicenter, placebo-controlled, double-blind trial of two doses (0.25 or 0.5 mg/day) of lasofoxifene compared to placebo for 5 years on the incidence of ER+ breast cancer in 8,556 postmenopausal women with low bone mass (osteopenia) on Dual Energy X ray Absorption (Hologic BMD T score −1.0 to −2.4) (Cummings et al. 2010; LaCroix et al. 2010). Participants had annual breast examination and mammography and breast cancers were confirmed by histopathology. The primary analysis was based on intent-to-treat using Cox Proportional Hazards models for breast cancers in each lasofoxifene group compared to placebo.

Breast cancer (invasive or noninvasive) occurred in 24 women in the placebo group compared to 20 women in the lasofoxifene 0.25 mg/day group (HR = 0.82, 95% CI 0.45–1.49, $p = 0.52$) and five women in the 0.5 mg/day lasofoxifene group (HR = 0.21, 95% CI 0.08–0.55 $p < 0.001$). ER-positive breast cancer (invasive or noninvasive) occurred in 21 women in the placebo group compared to 11 women in the lasofoxifene 0.25 mg/day group (HR = 0.52, 95%CI 0.25–1.08, $p = 0.073$) and four women in the 0.5 mg/day lasofoxifene group (HR = 0.19, 95% CI 0.07–0.56, $p < 0.001$). There was no reduction in ER-negative breast cancer. Lasofoxifene 0.5 mg/day caused a significant reduction in the incidence of vertebral fractures at 3 years (HR 0.58 95% CI 0.47–0.70) and nonvertebral fractures at 5 years (HR 0.76 95% CI 0.64–0.91). However, there was an increased risk of VTE events (HR 2.1 95% CI 1.20–3.60) but not stroke (HR 0.64 95% CI 0.41–0.99) and the incidence of major CHD events was significantly decreased (HR 0.68 95% CI 0.50–0.93). There was also an increase in gynecological toxicity including endometrial thickening, uterine polyps, and fibroids, but there was no increase in endometrial atypia or cancer. Overall mortality was similar for lasofoxifene 0.5 mg/day and placebo (HR 1.12 95% CI 0.80–1.56). In summary, 0.5 mg/day of lasofoxifene significantly reduced the incidence of ER-positive breast cancer, vertebral and non-vertebral fractures, and major coronary heart disease events with no detected increase in endometrial cancer risk in postmenopausal osteoporotic women.

12.4 Discussion

Both arzoxifene and lasofoxifene were developed primarily as osteoporosis drugs with breast cancer risk reduction as an added outcome. With so many effective drugs for treatment of osteoporosis, it is arguable that the emphasis should have been on developing a breast cancer risk-reducing SERM with added benefits compared to tamoxifen and raloxifene. The results from the PEARL trial reporting the spectrum of activity of lasofoxifene (0.5 mg/day) show that we have now probably achieved optimal development of SERMs, and further trials of SERMs are not planned. However, an important consideration which needs to be taken into account is that most of the side effects with tamoxifen occurs during treatment, whereas most of the cumulative benefit of breast cancer risk reduction occurs after treatment and continues for many years, perhaps a lifetime (Cuzick et al. 2007; Powles et al. 2007). This is likely to apply to all SERMs. Whether this optimization of the spectrum of benefits with low side effect profile will encourage more widespread use of SERMs to prevent breast cancer remains uncertain.

12

The main issue for acceptance of using SERMs for prevention of breast caner is the requirement of having to treat so many healthy women to prevent a relatively small number of cancers, even with the added benefits of reductions in fracture risk, major heart events, and stroke. This can only be resolved if we are able to identify those women who are likely to develop ER-positive breast cancer in order to take the strategy of SERM prevention of breast cancer forward to something that is clinically useful. At present we have no algorithm for predicting risk of ER-positive breast cancer. The Cambridge/Breast Cancer Association Consortium has identified single nucleotide polymorphisms (SNPs), which predict breast cancer risk, but their frequency in a normal population is quite low and not specific to ER-positive cancers (Shahana et al. 2009). It is possible that there are polymorphisms that are estrogen related which confer some advantages to the host such as increased fertility, better breast development for more successful lactation, etc. to account for a high frequency of occurrence. This may have been advantageous in earlier times but now that women live much longer predisposes to an increased breast cancer risk later. This inherent risk to ER-positive breast cancer could be exacerbated by interactions with environmental factors and may predispose to phenotypic features such as breast radiological density. With the currently available technology and with clinical specimens from the prevention trials, it should be possible to establish algorithms, which predict ER-positive breast cancer risk. Furthermore, we should be able to integrate these risk predictions into the risk factors for osteoporotic fractures, CHD, and stroke to identify a population of healthy women who may really gain overall clinical benefit from SERM intervention. This is likely to be possible once we are able to identify the commonly occurring SNPs, which predispose to these diseases, the interaction of environmental factor with the genetic risks, and the phenotypic features of these risk factors.

12.5 Conclusions

Clinical trials with SERMs have clearly shown that we can successfully prevent breast cancer in healthy women. Lasofoxifene 0.5 mg/day has been shown to have added benefits with reductions in the incidence of vertebral and nonvertebral fractures, major coronary heart events, and stroke. The challenge now is to identify those women who will benefit sufficiently from these treatments to justify use of such treatments in healthy women.

References

Baselga J, Llombart-Cussac A et al (2003) Randomized, double-blind, multicenter trial comparing two doses of arzoxifene (LY353381) in hormone-sensitive advanced or metastatic breast cancer patients. Ann Oncol 14:1383–1390

Buzdar A, O'Shaughnessy J et al (2003) Phase II randomized, double-blind study of two dose levels of arzoxifene in patients with locally advanced or metastatic breast cancer. J Clin Oncol 21(6):1007–1014

Cummings S, Norton L et al (1998) Raloxifene reduces the risk of breast cancer and may decrease the risk of endometrial cancer in postmenopausal women. Two-year findings from the multiple outcomes of raloxifene evaluation (MORE) trial. Proc Am Soc Clin Oncol 17:2a

Cummings S, Ensrud K et al (2010) Lasofoxifene in postmenopausal women with osteoporosis. N Engl J Med 362(8):686–696

Cuzick J, Forbes J et al (2002) First results from the International Breast Cancer Intervention Study (IBIS-I): a randomised prevention trial. Lancet 360:817–824

Cuzick J, Forbes J et al (2007) Long-term results of tamoxifen prophylaxis for breast cancer – 96 month follow-up of the randomised IBIS-I study. J Natl Cancer Inst 99:272–282

Deshmane V, Krishnamurthy S et al (2007) Phase III double-blind trial of arzoxifene compared with tamoxifen for locally advanced or metastatic breast cancer. J Clin Oncol 25(31):4967–4973

Fabian C, Kimler B et al (2004) Breast cancer chemoprevention phase I evaluation of biomarker modulation by arzoxifene, a third generation selective estrogen receptor modulator. Clin Cancer Res 10:5403–5417

Fisher B, Costantino J et al (1998) Tamoxifen for prevention of breast cancer: report of the National Surgical Adjuvant Breast and Bowel Project P-1 Study. JNCI 90(18):1371–1388

Ke H, Foley G et al (2004) Long-term treatment of lasofoxifene preserves bone mass and bone strength and does not adversely affect the uterus in ovariectomized rats. Endocrinology 145(4): 1996–2005

LaCroix A, Powles T et al (2010) "Breast cancer incidence in the PEARL trial of lasofoxifene in postmenopausal osteoporotic women." JNCI (in press)

McClung M, Siris E et al (2006) Prevention of bone loss in postmenopausal women treated with lasofoxifene compared with raloxifene. Menopause 13(3):325–327

Powles TJ, Ashley S et al (2007) "Twenty-Year follow-up of the royal marsden randomized double-blinded tamoxifen breast cancer prevention trial. J Natl Cancer Inst 99(4):283–290

Powles T, Diem S et al (2009) Effects of arzoxifene on breast cancer incidence in postmenopausal women with osteoporosis or with low bone mass (Abstract). San Antonio Breast Cancer Symposium, Texas, USA

Sato M, Turner C et al (1998) LY353381: a novel raloxifene analogue with improved SERM potency in vivo. Pharmacol Exp Ther 287:1–7

Shahana A, Thomas G et al (2009) Newly discovered breast cancer susceptibility loci on 3p24 and 17q23.2. Nat Genet 41:585–590

Suh N, Glasebrook A et al (2001) Arzoxifene, a new selective estrogen receptor modulator for chemoprevention of experimental breast cancer. Cancer Res 61(23):8412–8415

Vogel V, Costantino J et al (2006) Effects of tamoxifen vs raloxifene on the risk of developing invasive breast cancer and other disease outcomes – the NSABP study of tamoxifen and raloxifene (STAR) P-2 trial. JAMA 295: 2727–2741

13 Chemoprevention of Hormone Receptor-Negative Breast Cancer: New Approaches Needed

Iván P. Uray and Powel H. Brown

Abstract Results from clinical trials have demonstrated that it is possible to prevent estrogen-responsive breast cancers by targeting the estrogen receptor with selective estrogen receptor modulators (SERMs) (tamoxifen, raloxifene, or lasofoxifene) or with aromatase inhibitors (AIs) (anastrozole, letrozole, or exemestene). Results from breast cancer treatment trials suggest that aromatase inhibitors may be even more effective in preventing breast cancer than SERMs. However, while SERMs and aromatase inhibitors do prevent the development of many ER-positive breast cancers, these drugs do not prevent ER-negative breast cancer. These results show that new approaches are needed for the prevention of this aggressive form of breast cancer. Our laboratory and clinical efforts have been focused on identifying critical molecular pathways in breast cells that can be targeted for the prevention of ER-negative breast cancer. Our preclinical studies have demonstrated that other nuclear receptors, such as RXR receptors, vitamin D receptors, as well as others are critical for the growth of ER-negative breast cells and for the transformation of these cells into ER-negative cancers. Other studies show that growth factor pathways including those activated by EGFR, Her2, and IGFR, which are activated in many ER-negative breast cancers, can be targeted for the prevention of ER-negative breast cancer in mice. Clinical studies have also shown that PARP inhibitors are effective for the treatment of breast cancers arising in BRCA-1 or -2 mutation carriers, suggesting that targeting PARP may also be useful for the prevention of breast cancers arising in these high-risk individuals. Most recently, we have demonstrated that ER-negative breast cancers can be subdivided into four distinct groups based on the kinases that they express. These groups include ER-negative/Her-2-positive groups (the MAPK and immunomodulatory groups) and ER-negative/Her2-negative groups (the S6K and the cell cycle checkpoint groups). These groups of ER-negative breast cancers can be targeted with kinase inhibitors specific for each subgroup. These preclinical studies have supported the development of several clinical trials testing targeted agents for the prevention of breast cancer. The results of a completed Phase II cancer prevention trial using the RXR ligand bexarotene in women at

I.P. Uray and P.H. Brown (✉)
Department of Clinical Cancer Prevention,
The University of Texas M. D. Anderson Cancer Center, 1155 Herman P. Pressler, Unit 1360,
Houston, TX 77230, USA
e-mail: phbrown@mdanderson.org

H.-J. Senn and F. Otto (eds.), *Clinical Cancer Prevention*,
Recent Results in Cancer Research 188, DOI: 10.1007/978-3-642-10858-7_13,

13

high risk of breast cancer will be reviewed, and the current status of an ongoing Phase II trial using the EGFR and Her2 kinase inhibitor lapatinib for the treatment of women with DCIS breast cancer will be presented. It is anticipated that in the future these molecularly targeted drugs will be combined with hormonal agents such as SERMs or aromatase inhibitors to prevent all forms of breast cancer.

This work was supported by NCI/NIH Grants RO1 CA10121, RO1 CA78480, and a PROMISE grant from the Susan G. Komen for the Cure Foundation.

While the action of antiestrogenic drugs used for cancer prevention is relatively well understood and improved pharmacologic agents are being developed, it is important to look for alternative molecular mechanisms by which biologically active chemical compounds can effectively reduce the incidence of breast cancer, regardless of the tissues' estrogen receptor status. This review will present the directions taken by current investigations to identify viable candidate drugs categorized by their mechanisms of action, and shed new insights into off-label applications of currently used therapeutics.

13.1 Introduction

In the year 2009 over 190,000 new cases of breast cancer were diagnosed and approximately 40,000 deaths from breast cancer have occurred in the United States (Horner et al. 2009). Current strategies using endocrine agents have successfully prevented or treated estrogen receptor-positive breast cancers by interfering with estrogen signaling or production. The model-selective estrogen receptor modulator (SERM), tamoxifen, and another, less toxic antiestrogen drug, raloxifene, have been shown to prevent estrogen receptor-positive breast cancer in high-risk women (Fisher et al. 1998; Cummings et al. 1999; Cuzick et al. 2003). However, these drugs only reduced breast cancer incidence by 50%, and had no effect on preventing estrogen receptor-negative breast cancer, which accounts for 30% of all breast cancers (Fisher et al. 1998; Vogel et al. 2006). These factors make the compelling case that novel agents need to be discovered that will aid in the prevention and/or treatment of estrogen receptor-negative breast cancer.

13.2 Endocrine Preventive Agents

In recent years, significant progress has been made in demonstrating that drugs targeted against the estrogen receptor, such as selective estrogen receptor modulators (SERMs) and aromatase inhibitors, are useful for the treatment and prevention of breast cancer.

13.3 Selective Estrogen Receptor Modulators

A host of preclinical models have been used over the years to demonstrate that estrogen is a key factor for the initiation and promotion of breast cancer, suggesting a potential therapeutic and preventive effect for antiestrogenic agents (Fig. 13.1). It has been established early on that pregnancy can promote, and bilateral oophorectomy is protective against breast cancer development. The accumulating knowledge of estrogen signaling and the identification of estrogen receptor ultimately led to the design of drugs targeting the estrogen receptor (Lerner et al. 1958). The

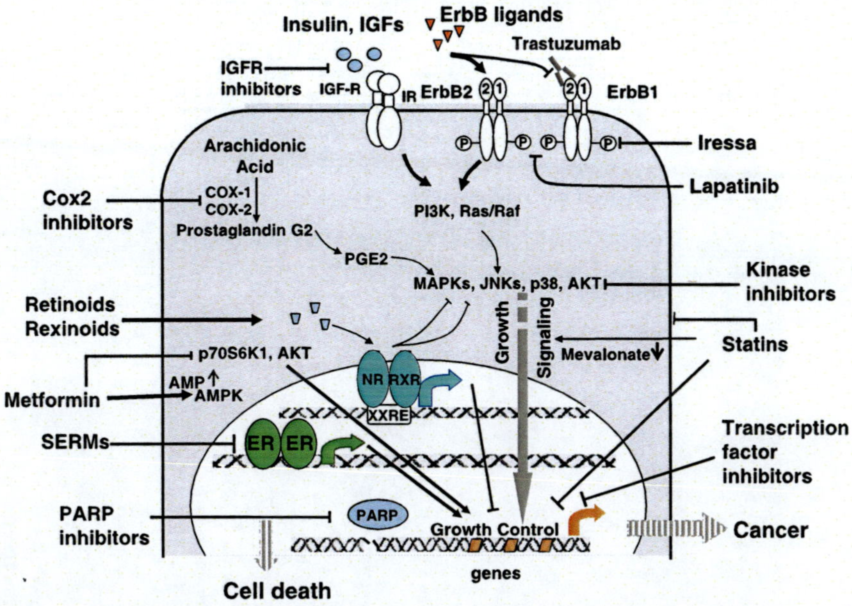

Fig. 13.1 Pathways to target for the prevention of breast cancer. Estrogen-dependent (via the estrogen receptor alpha) and estrogen-independent pathways are shown

first group of compounds that were used to suppress ER signaling are SERMs, compounds exhibiting selective agonistic or antagonistic properties depending on the target tissue. The first antiestrogenic agent to be approved for the treatment and ultimately for the prevention of breast cancer was tamoxifen (Honig 2001). Tamoxifen competitively inhibits binding of estrogen to ER and therefore is an antagonist of estrogenic signaling in breast tissue, but acts as an agonist in bone and the uterus. In several adjuvant studies, tamoxifen was found to significantly reduce the incidence of contralateral breast cancer as an endpoint (Cuzick and Baum 1985). This observation implicated the chemopreventive effect of tamoxifen in healthy women at high risk of breast cancer and led to a series of cancer prevention trials.

A comprehensive meta-analysis summarizing all tamoxifen prevention trials concluded that the overall reduction in breast cancer incidence by tamoxifen was 38% (95% CI, 28–46, $p < 0.001$, Table 13.1) (Cuzick et al. 2003). Tamoxifen over 5 years reduced the frequency of new ER-positive breast cancers by 48%, and long-term follow-up of the IBIS-I trial suggests that the risk-reducing effect of tamoxifen persists for at least 10 years, while most side effects of tamoxifen do not continue after the 5-year treatment period (Cuzick et al. 2007). In all these studies, tamoxifen had no effect on the development of ER-negative breast cancers (Fisher et al. 2005; Powles et al. 2007; Cummings et al. 1999; Cuzick et al. 2007; Veronesi et al. 2007). Apart from its benefits, long-term tamoxifen treatment was associated with side effects, including increased risk of endometrial cancer, venous thromboembolism, and hot flushes, which were observed in all studies. Concerns about tamoxifen-related toxicity, that limited its use as a preventive agent, became the driving force to identify novel

Table 13.1 Status of phase III breast cancer prevention trials

Trial	Phase III breast cancer prevention trials of SERMs or aromatase inhibitors					
	Intervention	Sample size	Patient eligibility	Endpoints	Results	Reference
NSABP-P1	Placebo vs tamoxifen, 20 mg	13,388	>1.6% 5-year risk	Incidence of IBC	49% Reduction in breast cancer	Fisher et al. (2005)
Royal Marsden Hospital	Placebo vs tamoxifen, 20 mg	2,494	High-risk, family history	Incidence of IBC	Negative at 5 years; significantly lower risk of ER+ BC in the posttreatment (>8 years) period	Powles et al. (2007)
Italian breast cancer prevention trial with tamoxifen	Placebo vs tamoxifen, 20 mg	5,408	Normal-risk, hysterectomy	Incidence of IBC	Reduction of IBC in patients starting HRT after tamoxifen	Veronesi et al. (2007)
IBIS-I	Placebo vs tamoxifen, 20 mg	7,152	>2-fold relative risk, healthy	Frequency of IBC or DCIS	31% Reduction in invasive ER-positive tumors	Cuzick et al. (2007)
MORE	Placebo vs raloxifen, 60 mg or 120 mg	7,705	Normal-risk, postmenopausal women with osteoporosis	Fracture risk, breast cancer	76% Reduction in the risk of IBC during 3 years	Cummings et al. (1999)
NSABP STAR	Tamoxifen, 20 mg vs raloxifene 60 mg	19,747	≥1.7% 5-year risk	Incidence of IBC	No difference (estimated a 50% reduction by both)	Vogel et al. (2006)
PEARL	Calcium + vitamin D, plus placebo vs 0.25–0.5 mg lasofoxifene	8,556	Women age 59–80, negative mammography, bone mineral density T score <-2.5	Bone fractures, ER+ BC, coronary heart disease, stroke	Reduced risk of fractures, ER-positive breast cancer, coronary heart disease, stroke	Cummings (2010)
IBIS-II Prevention	Placebo vs anastrozole, 1 mg	6,000 (planned)	Postmenopausal, high risk	Frequency of BC, both invasive and noninvasive	Earliest results in 2012	Cuzick (2008)
IBIS-II DCIS	Placebo vs anastrozole or tamoxifen	4,000 (planned)	Postmenopausal, prior ER+ DCIS	Incidence of new cancer in affected and contralateral breast	Earliest results in 2012	Cuzick (2003, 2008)
MAP.3	Placebo vs exemestane, 25 mg	4,560	Postmenopausal, 5-year risk >1.67% based on Gail model	Frequency of invasive BC	Trial ongoing	Goss et al. (2007)

SERMs with less toxicity and resulted in the development of raloxifene and lasofoxifene for clinical use.

The Study of Tamoxifen and Raloxifene (STAR) trial demonstrated that raloxifene was equivalent to tamoxifen in its ability to decrease the risk of breast cancer in high-risk postmenopausal women, but patients taking raloxifene had less toxicity, uterine cancers, and blood clots than those who received tamoxifen (Vogel et al. 2006). In 2007 in the United States, raloxifene received FDA approval for preventive use in postmenopausal women with osteoporosis or at high risk for invasive breast cancer. A more recently developed nonsteroidal SERM lasofoxifene exhibited a better toxicity profile in postmenopausal women with osteoporosis. As recently published results of the PEARL trial show, lasofoxifene (given at 0.5 mg/day for 5 years) reduced the incidence of ER-positive breast tumors (invasive and noninvasive) by 81% in postmenopausal women with osteoporosis. As primary end point the study also established that lasofoxifene reduced the risk of both vertebral and nonvertebral bone fractures and coronary disease, but increased the risk of venous thromboembolic events (Cummings et al. 2010).

13.4 Aromatase Inhibitors

Aromatase inhibitors present an alternative strategy to antagonize estrogen-dependent signaling by blocking the biosynthesis of estrogen through reversible (nonsteroidal agents such as letrozole and anastrozole) or irreversible (steroidal agents, i.e., exemestane) inhibition of the aromatase enzyme (Fig. 13.1). AIs have proven an effective approach to treatment of existing breast cancers in premenopausal women. Their chemopreventive potential was first identified in adjuvant studies, yet so far no AI has been fully evaluated for cancer-preventive use.

In animals and in humans AIs performed better than tamoxifen in potency and response duration to cause regression of breast tumors. Similarly, hypothesis-generating adjuvant trials involving AIs (ATAC, MA.17 and IES testing anastrazole, letrozole or exemestane, respectively) showed that the tested agents were more effective than tamoxifen to delay the recurrence of a prior breast cancer or prevent second primary cancers (Cuzick 2003; Goss et al. 2007). In addition, fewer thromboembolic events and endometrial cancers were reported following AI treatment, although the risk of fractures and arthralgias was increased with AI use (Chlebowski et al. 2009). Similarly, the MA.17 and MAP.3 trials have shown that switching from tamoxifen to letrozole or exemestane, respectively, reduced the risk of a contralateral formation of breast cancer in ER-positive patients. Studies on the long-term outcomes of the ATAC trial provided evidence of a larger carryover effect after 5 years of adjuvant treatment with anastrozole compared with tamoxifen (Forbes et al. 2008).

Meta-analyses of AI monotherapy and sequenced therapy (tamoxifen switched to AI) clinical trials showed that disease-free survival was significantly improved for both options and overall survival was prolonged for patients who switched from tamoxifen to AI therapy (Josefsson and Leinster 2010).

Based on the experience of the ATAC trial, the Breast International Group (BIG) proposed and is conducting the IBIS-II Prevention (high-risk portion of IBIS-II) trial, which will determine the cancer-preventive effect of anastrozole versus placebo in postmenopausal women at increased risk of breast cancer. The primary endpoint is the frequency of invasive and noninvasive breast cancer. A parallel randomized phase III trial termed IBIS-II – DCIS, is comparing anastrozole against tamoxifen in 4,000 women with locally excised DCIS

(Cuzick 2008; Dunn and Ryan 2009). The primary endpoints are the comparison of the efficacy of adjuvant tamoxifen versus anastrozole in local control and prevention of contralateral disease, as well as the comparison of side effects.

In spite of promising results seen with AIs as chemopreventive agents, AIs can only be used in postmenopausal women and are not expected to suppress ER-negative breast cancer incidence. Thus, the prevention of receptor-negative breast cancer requires the identification of novel mechanisms that target nonestrogen signaling pathways.

13.5 New Strategies to Prevent Hormone-Independent Breast Cancer

13.5.1 PARP Inhibitors

The use of poly(ADP-ribose) polymerase (PARP) inhibitors constitutes a novel approach to targeted cancer therapy. Cells carrying heterozygous loss-of-function mutations of BRCA may lose the wild-type allele on the path of oncogenesis, making these cells deficient in their ability of homologous recombination. In the absence of PARP1, spontaneous single-strand breaks collapse DNA replication forks and trigger homologous recombination for repair, making any DNA damage lethal to the BRCA mutant cell. Bryant and collagues have elegantly shown that BRCA2-deficient cells, as a result of their deficiency in homologous recombination, are acutely sensitive to PARP inhibitors (Bryant et al. 2005). The requirement of a BRCA mutation to be present for a PARP inhibitor to be effective constitutes a "synthetic lethal" strategy selectively affecting BRCA1 or 2 mutant tumor cells (a compound targeting a particular pathway is selectively "lethal" to cells harboring a mutation in a complementary pathway).

Based on encouraging preclinical studies, Phase I clinical trials (NCI-08-C-0128, NCI-09-C-0048) were initiated, which assessed the safety, tolerability of the PARP inhibitors AZD2281, and ABT-888 in combination with DNA-damaging chemotherapeutic drugs cisplatin and gemcitabine. PARP inhibitors were scored based on PARP activity (formation of poly(ADP-ribose) moieties and γH2AX foci), DNA damage, cell proliferation, and cell death. The single agent Phase I clinical evaluation (NCT00516373) of the orally active PARP inhibitor olaparib (4-[(3-{[4-cyclopropylcarbonyl)piperazin-1-yl]carbonyl}-4-fluorophenyl)methyl]phthalazin-1(2H)-one), or AZD2281, has been recently completed and reported few of the adverse effects of conventional chemotherapy (Fong et al. 2009). A multicenter, single-arm phase II study of contiuous oral olaparib in BRCA1/BRCA2 carriers with recurrent, chemotherapy-refractory breast cancers provided a positive proof of concept, as olaparib at 400 mg bd was well tolerated and highly active (Tutt et al. 2009). Toxicity was reported as mainly mild, symptoms included fatigue (33%), nausea (27%), vomiting (15%), and anemia (4%). Given the relatively good tolerability profile of PARP inhibitors, these agents may be well suited for cancer-preventive use. Since the inhibition of a DNA repair enzyme in the absence of an exogenous DNA-damaging agent is sufficient to selectively kill tumor cells while posing no threat to normal cells, PARP inhibitors could present themselves as the ideal chemopreventive strategy. To further investigate their clinical applicability as chemopreventive agents, further investigations should be proposed in BRCA mutation carriers to assess the ability of PARP inhibitors of reducing the incidence of breast cancer.

13.6 Cell Growth Inhibitors

13.6.1 Statins

Statins potently inhibit cholesterol biosynthesis by blocking the production of mevalonate and therefore have been in clinical use as lipid-lowering drugs for over 30 years. In addition to reducing sterol biosynthesis, statins may interfere with microdomain formation, improve endothelial function by interfering with oxidative stress pathways (Mason et al. 2004). While their beneficial effects on mortality from cardiovascular disease have been well documented, the prospect of statins' utility as a cancer-preventive drug remains controversial. There is strong preclinical evidence to suggest that lipophilic statins, atorvastatin, lovastatin, simvastatin, and fluvastatin significantly inhibit the proliferation of breast cancer cell lines, and greater suppression was observed in ER-negative cell lines (Mueck et al. 2003). In addition, fluvastatin, simvastatin, and lovastatin, but not pravastatin, have been shown to possess growth inhibitory activities at therapeutic doses in ER-negative mouse breast cancer models (Campbell et al. 2006). However, epidemiologic studies have resulted in mixed conclusions. Kumar and coworkers have found a marked reduction of breast cancers associated with the administration of lipophilic statins (Kumar et al. 2006). In addition, breast cancer patients on long-term statin treatment have proportionately fewer ER/PR-negative tumors that are of lower grade and stage, than patients who never received statins (Kumar et al. 2008). On the other hand, Bonovas and coworkers concluded from a meta-analysis of seven randomized and nine observational breast cancer trials that statin use did not significantly affect breast cancer risk (Bonovas et al. 2005). Similar statistical evaluations were carried out by this group retrospectively to assess the cancer-preventive effects of statins against a number of other cancers, including prostate, colon, and skin, with similar negative results. However, such meta-analyses of randomized trials were criticized on the basis of including both lipophilic and nonlipophilic statin use. It was also argued that these trials were originally designed and the dosages set up with respect to cardiovascular endpoints, and so conclusions on breast cancer risk may be misleading.

Several phase II prevention trials are ongoing at the NCI using lipophilic statins (JHOC-J0485, V0407, BRSNSTU0010), to assess their cancer-preventive effects using biomarkers. Most recently a perioperative window trial was carried out focusing on the cancer-preventive effects of only fluvastatin in women with a diagnosis of DCIS or stage 1 breast cancer. The investigators reported measurable biologic changes with reduced tumor proliferation and increased apoptotic activity (Garwood et al. 2010). Since these effects were evident only in high-grade, very early-stage tumors, these results call for further evaluation of statins as chemopreventive agents for ER-negative high-grade breast cancers.

13.6.2 Metformin

Several studies have identified an increased risk of cancer in noninsulin-dependent diabetics (Xue and Michels 2007). A recent meta-analysis of 20 studies of breast cancer has confirmed the long-time notion that there is increased risk of breast cancer associated with diabetes (Larsson et al. 2007). It was suggested that insulin may activate various proliferative and antiapoptotic mechanisms leading to or promoting carcinogenesis (Papa and Belfiore 1996). Therefore, the question as to whether the lowering of insulin levels by antidiabetic therapy would decrease cancer incidence or cancer mortality merits investigation (Goodwin 2008).

13

Experimental studies have found that in carcinogen-treated mice or in tumor-prone transgenic mice exercise reduces the odds for the development of cancer. Studies in animal models have shown that AMP kinase activators such as phenformin, metformin, and AICAR inhibit tumor development. Furthermore, in vitro studies in epithelial cells have demonstrated that metformin activates the cellular energy sensor AMP kinase through the tumor suppressor LKB1, whose genetic loss is associated with Peutz-Jeghers syndrome and increased risk of epithelial cancers (Giardiello et al. 2000). Enzymes inhibited by AMPK include mammalian homolog of Target Of Rapamycin (mTOR), acetyl-CoA carboxylase (ACC), fatty acid synthase (FAS), and glycerol phosphate acyltransferase (GPAT) – key regulators of protein, fatty acid, and glycerolipid syntheses. Multiple metabolic pathways indicating energy saturation (leptin, adiponectin, IL6, resveratrol) converge onto AMPK to induce downregulation of glycogen, fatty acid, and cholesterol synthesis. In addition, AMPK activation suppresses cell growth through the inhibition of protein synthesis and the upregulation of the p53 pathway resulting in the induction of p21, reduction of cyclin D1 levels, and cell cycle arrest (Zakikhani et al. 2006).

Metformin is a biguanide derivative approved for the treatment of type II diabetes mellitus, with antihyperglycemic properties. The prevailing view on the action of metformin is the reduction of hepatic glucose output by inhibition of gluconeogenesis, with resulting suppression of insulin levels (Shaw et al. 2005), but it is also thought to increase sensitivity of peripheral tissues to insulin (Bailey and Turner 1996). Whether a possible cancer-preventive effect can be attributed to this systemic effect or to a direct growth suppressive effect of metformin remains unclear. However, it has also been proposed that metformin by activating AMPK may be able to overcome breast cancer resistance to Her2 inhibitors while decreasing risk of cardiotoxicity (Vazquez-Martin et al. 2009).

The European Institute of Oncology in Milan is currently conducting a two-arm Phase II clinical trial testing metformin against placebo in women with early breast cancer. This presurgical randomized, double blind, placebo-controlled biomarker trial will enroll 100 histologically confirmed breast cancer patients and use metformin at 850 mg twice daily for 28 + 7 days before surgery, to assess drug activity. The primary endpoint of the study is the change in tumor and dysplastic/hyperplastic cell proliferation, as measured by the percentage of Ki67 positive cells (Cazzaniga et al. 2009). A successful outcome could pave the way for a subsequent chemoprevention trial with metformin (Goodwin et al. 2009).

The use of metformin for cancer prevention could be perceived as a paradigm shift in the drug development process. Because the same pathway may be involved in different tumors and in different diseases, molecularly targeted agents, which target pathways instead of diseases could present a better approach than the "one disease, one drug model."

13.6.3 Retinoids

Retinoids, derivatives of vitamin A, are small, lipophilic molecules with pleiotropic effects on development, differentiation, and homeostatic regulation of most tissues (Szanto et al. 2004). Several lines of evidence from in vitro systems suggest that retinoids may control various mechanisms directly or indirectly suppressing cell growth, independent of the ER/PR status of the cell. We and others have shown that retinoids induce G1 cell cycle arrest, overexpression of the IGF binding proteins 3 and 6, RARβ, TGFβ, and down-regulate COX-2 and cyclin D1 expression, as well as inhibit the activity of the AP-1 transcription factor (Lee et al. 1996; Seewaldt et al. 1997; Yang et al. 2001; Kong et al. 2005; Wu et al. 2006; Uray et al. 2009).

Cancer prevention using specific compounds traces back to the early twentieth century when Wolbach first reported on his rat study with "tissue changes following deprivation of fat-soluble A vitamin" and the reverse changes that follow, when the rats are restored to an adequate diet (Wolbach and Howe 1925). Although there is little epidemiologic data supporting the use of vitamin A or carotenoids to reduce breast cancer risk, the ability of retinoids to prevent cancer was demonstrated later in various animal models. Retinyl acetate, and the synthetic retinoid N-(4-hydroxyphenyl) retinamide (4-HPR) have been used to prevent mammary carcinogenesis in rats exposed to chemical carcinogens (Moon et al. 1979). The naturally occurring 9-cis-RA was also found to suppress mammary tumors alone or in combination with low-dose tamoxifen (Wu et al. 2000; Anzano et al. 1994).

One of the first reports on molecular-targeted chemoprevention research demonstrated that an adjuvant high dose of isotretinoin (13-*cis*-retinoic acid) prevented second primary tumors in patients with curatively treated head and neck cancer (Hong et al. 1990). While this was a seminal discovery, which greatly helped establish translational retinoid research, the toxicity of this retinoid has prevented its general clinical use. Another naturally occurring retinoid 9-*cis*-retinoic acid (9cRA) reduces the incidence of mammary tumors, but it also induces liver toxicity, hair loss, and skin erythema (Wu et al. 2000).

While retinoids can only bind retinoic acid receptors, a special class of retinoids termed rexinoids activates hetero- or homodimers of the retinoid X receptor (RXR). The fact that RXRs are potential dimerization partners of a number of nuclear hormone receptors, such as RARs, VDR, TRs, PPARs, and others, yields a highly flexible and complex signaling system, able to induce gene expression characteristic of other partners. However, the composition of the nuclear receptor heterodimers that mediate the cancer-preventive effect of retinoids and rexinoids is unknown and is under investigation in our laboratory. Our laboratory and others have shown that retinoid X receptor-selective drugs (rexinoids) prevent breast cancer in mice more effectively and with less toxicity than retinoids. Specifically, the synthetic rexinoids bexarotene and LG100268 have been shown to prevent estrogen receptor-negative breast cancer in various mouse models including transgenic lines of MMTV-ErbB2 overexpressing, p53-null, and C3(1)-SV40 T-antigen (Tag) expressing mice and rats (Wu et al. 2002a, b; Liby et al. 2008; Medina et al. 2009; Woditschka et al. 2006). In addition, we have shown that LGD100268 significantly prevents premalignant lesions including hyperplasia and ductal carcinoma in situ, suggesting that it affects mammary tumorigenesis at the early stages (Li et al. 2007).

The effectiveness of bexarotene to prevent breast cancer formation in humans may be accompanied by mild hyperlipidemia, skin rash, hypothyroidism, elevated liver enzymes, and neutropenia (at high doses only). The positive data from the preclinical studies provided the rationale to launch a human biomarker modulation trial using bexarotene in women at high risk of breast cancer in a 4-week period. This trial has determined that bexarotene significantly down-regulates cyclin D1 expression and decreases proliferation, as measured by Ki67 staining (this latter change did not reach statistical significance) (as presented in abstract form at the 2008 AACR Frontiers in Cancer Prevention Symposium). Interestingly, these responses occurred selectively in postmenopausal women. The results from this trial will provide a reference for other rexinoids to develop more effective and safer preventive drugs.

Combination treatment may represent a promising new strategy to suppress both ER-negative and ER-positive breast tumors, and the combination of rexinoids with antiestrogens may be particularly effective. Recent studies reported on the highly synergistic effect of the RXR agonist LGD100268 and the selective estrogen receptor modulator arzoxifene through the inhibition of cell growth and induction of apoptosis (Rendi et al. 2004; Liby et al. 2006). Early results from our ongoing animal experiments also indicate that tamoxifen used in combination with bexarotene or LG100268 is superior to either drug alone.

13.6.4 PPAR Agonists

Peroxisome proliferator-activated receptors (PPAR) are members of the nuclear hormone receptor superfamily selectively modulating the expression of their target genes forming heterodimers with RXRs. PPARγ plays an important role in adipocyte differentiation, insulin sensitivity, energy metabolism, and immune response. Recently, PPARγ has emerged as a promising target for cancer therapy based on the fact that its activation by synthetic ligands, thiazolidinediones (TZDs), was found to induce cell cycle arrest, apoptosis, and differentiation in human malignancies (Mueller et al. 1998; Yin et al. 2001). Troglitazone, a PPARγ ligand, induced apoptosis in both ER-positive and ER-negative human breast cancer cells (Clay et al. 1999; Yin et al. 2004). Activation of PPARγ by the antidiabetic drug rosiglitazone caused tumor-selective suppression of the NHE1 transporter and inhibition of cancer cell proliferation in vitro and in pathologic specimens from breast cancer patients (Kumar et al. 2009). The chemopreventive potential of PPARγ was demonstrated in experimental rodent mammary tumorigenesis models (Suh et al. 1999), as the PPARγ ligand GW7845 significantly reduced tumor incidence, multiplicity, and weight. Similarly, troglitazone prevented the development of DMBA-induced premalignant lesions in mouse mammary organ culture (Mehta et al. 2000). Natural occurring ligands such as conjugated linoleic acids may be regarded as a component of the diet that exert antineoplastic activity and its effect have also been found to inhibit progression of mammary tumorigenesis (Ip et al. 1999; Maggiora et al. 2004; Wendel and Heller 2009). These data suggested that PPAR ligands maybe useful in preventing the development of ER-negative breast cancers.

13.6.5 COX-2 Inhibitors

There is a wealth of epidemiological data to suggest that long-term use of aspirin or nonsteroidal antiinflammatory drugs (NSAIDs) is associated with a reduced risk of various cancers, in particular of the digestive system (Schreinemachers and Everson 1994). The biochemical effect of NSAIDs is the inhibition of cyclooxigenase (COX) enzymes, which play a crucial role in growth-promoting prostaglandin synthesis via the eicosanoid pathway (Fig. 13.1). Overexpression of the inducible isoform COX-2 has been demonstrated for several human cancers including, breast, lung, esophageal, hepatocellular, and most notably colorectal adenocarcinomas (Turini and DuBois 2002). It has also been suggested that there is cross talk between COX-2 and EGFR via MAPK signaling resulting in the induction of the COX-2 enzyme, which underscores the rationale for combination chemoprevention (Dannenberg et al. 2005). Meta-analysis on cohort and case–control studies has revealed that NSAID use may also be associated with a small decrease in the risk of breast cancer (Khuder and Mutgi 2001).

Multiple studies have tested the cancer-preventive effect of various NSAIDs and selective COX-2 inhibitors in animal models. Celecoxib, a selective COX-2 inhibitor, reduced the incidence and multiplicity of DMBA-induced mammary tumors in rat models by 68% and 86%, respectively (Harris et al. 2000). In MMTV-erbB2 transgenic mice, which mainly develop ER-negative cancers, celecoxib at 500 ppm delayed mammary tumor development and decreased the levels of PGE2 by 50%, suggesting that COX-2 inhibitors might be able to prevent ER-negative breast cancer (Howe et al. 2002). Conversely, other studies suggest that COX-2 might not be the only or ideal target in the eicosanoid pathway (Rigas and Kashfi 2005). This notion is supported by the facts that COX-2 is induced at a relatively later stage in carcinogenesis, NSAIDs may not require inhibition of COX-2 for their effect, and lastly, NSAIDs have a modest effect in the preventive setting.

There is a concern that inhibition of COX-2 in nonneoplastic cell might be harmful and cause unwanted toxicity. Indeed, phase III polyp prevention trials of COX-2 inhibitors uncovered rare, late, but serious cardiovascular toxicities of these drugs. In response to an increase in the risk of heart attacks observed in individuals taking celecoxib the FDA temporarily halted all ongoing celecoxib trials, including those for breast cancer prevention. Later the trials were allowed to continue, but these rare and serious side effects likely will limit the widespread use of COX-2 inhibitors as cancer prevention agents. However, use in populations at low risk for heart disease may be found to be safe and effective. Interfering with PGE2-induced signaling by targeting prostanoid (EP) receptors, such as EP4 or downstream targets, may also offer a safer alternative to COX-2 inhibition.

13.6.6 Tyrosine Kinase Inhibitors

13.6.6.1 The erbB System

Epithelial cells largely depend on extracellular growth signals transmitted by receptor tyrosine kinases (see Fig. 13.1). Epidermal and other growth factors trigger autophosphorylation of their receptors, which in turn initiates a cascade of signaling events involving the activation of the ras pathway kinases via Grb2/SOS and MAPK activation. These mitogenic signaling events result in the activation of cell cycle genes and inhibition of programmed cell death. Overexpression of the MAP kinases p44 Erk1 and p42 Erk2 have also been shown in human breast tumors (Salh et al. 1999).

Breast cancers often arise from aberrant expression or activation of the erbB family of growth factor receptors (Hynes and Lane 2005), consisting of four distinct members, epidermal growth factor receptor (EGFR, erbB1or Her-1), erbB2 (Her2 or neu), erbB3 (Her-3), and erbB4 (Her4). 20–30% of all human mammary tumors, particularly those that are ER-negative, overexpress the erbB2 oncogene or one of its homologues (Ariga et al. 2005). The EGFR mediates the actions of a family of growth factors, which includes EGF, transforming growth factor alpha, and the neuregulins.

The usefulness of TKIs for the treatment of cancer has been indicated by studies of imatinib mesylate (STI-571/Gleevec), a cAbl, and c-kit tyrosine kinase inhibitor that was used successfully for the treatment of chronic myelogenous leukemia and gastrointestinal stromal tumors (Savage and Antman 2002; Sawyers et al. 2002). Several different signaling inhibitors that block the activity of the ErbB family of receptors have been developed and approved for clinical use, including herceptin (Trastuzumab), gefitinib (Iressa), and erlotinib (Tarceva). Herceptin, a humanized monoclonal Her-2 antibody, is highly effective for the treatment Her-2-positive breast cancers, but antibody treatment may not be viable in the prevention setting. In preclinical models we have demonstrated that gefitinib prevents the development of ER-negative mammary tumors (Lu et al. 2003) and others have shown that it is superior to herceptin in suppressing growth of DCIS epithelial cells (Chan et al. 2001). Gefitinib was released for phase II and III testing for the treatment of lung, prostate, and breast cancer, and is now approved for the treatment of lung cancer. However, due to the onset of pulmonary fibrosis as a rare side effect attributed to the drug all cancer-preventive trials using gefitinib were put on hold.

Both in vitro and in vivo studies demonstrated that dual inhibition of EGFR and Her-2 more effectively suppresses cell growth and survival than the inhibition of either receptor alone (Moulder et al. 2001), prompting the development of multivalent erbB receptor inhibitors. A number of new EGFR-selective (PD153035, AG1478, AG1517, PD158780, PD165557, PKI 166) and multitarget (lapatinib, HKI-272, BIBW-2992, BMS-599626, targeting EGFR and Her-2; CI-1033 targeting EGFR, Her-2 and erbB4) inhibitors have been developed and are now in clinical testing for the treatment of various solid tumors.

Lapatinib (Tykerb®, GlaxoSmithKline) was first approved to use in combination with capecitabine (Xeloda), for women whose breast cancer had progressed on previous chemotherapies. Lapatinib had similar activity in HER2-positive breast tumors as a monotherapy or in combination with capecitabine. In early 2010, the US Food and Drug Administration granted approval to lapatinib for use in combination with the aromatase inhibitor letrozole for the treatment of postmenopausal women with hormone receptor positive metastatic breast cancer that overexpresses the Her-2 receptor and for whom hormonal therapy is indicated. Based on the results of the randomized phase III study EGF30008 the European Medicines Agency also issued its positive opinion for the authorization of lapatinib in combination with letrozole.

Our group has shown that lapatinib significantly delays breast cancer development in MMTV-erbB2 transgenic mice and prevents the development of premalignant mammary lesions (Strecker et al. 2009). These results suggest that lapatinib may be a good candidate as a cancer-preventive agent and the first neoadjuvant trial has begun in women with DCIS breast cancer in a multicenter clinical trial.

13.6.7 The IGF System

Insulin-like growth factors play a pertinent role in the growth regulation of mammary epithelial cells. IGF-I is bound with high affinity by type I insulin-like growth factor receptor (IGF-IR) and activates cellular proliferation in both normal growth and development and malignant transformation. IGF-I signals are mediated via phosphorylation of a family of insulin receptor substrate proteins (IRS), which may serve both complementary and overlapping functions to insulin receptor (IR) in the cell.

In addition to the important role of the IGF system in normal mammary development, it has been proposed that overproduction of GH or IGF-I can also cause the development of atypical hyperplasias or even carcinoma (Kleinberg et al. 2009). While it is not understood how early full-term pregnancy can provide natural protection against breast cancer, serum GH levels, and downstream signaling activity were shown to be decreased in parous animals compared to virgins (Dearth et al. 2010). Therefore, novel agents targeting the GH/IGF-I axis may provide a viable means to block formation and progression of neoplastic precursor lesions. As a proof of principle, the new IGF-IR tyrosine kinase inhibitor, BMS-536924 caused a blockade of cell proliferation in monolayer and 3D cell cultures, and reversed the ability of constitutively active IGF-IR to transform MCF10A cells (Litzenburger et al. 2009). Thus, agents known to block mammary gland development through inhibition of IGF-I action, may also present themselves as candidates for chemoprevention in women at high risk of breast cancer.

13.6.8 Conclusions and Future Directions

Since Michael Sporn introduced the term “chemoprevention” in the 1970s, the breast cancer prevention field has taken unexpected directions and is now facing new challenges. Firstly, while clinical trials have demonstrated that antiestrogen drug treatment of high-risk women can prevent breast cancer, there has not been widespread use of these drugs for cancer prevention.

In addition, the testing of new preventive drugs has been slow and costly. To increase the success rate of future clinical cancer prevention research, it will be necessary to conduct many small-scale, phase 0, I, and II trials focused on high-risk women. Target populations should be carefully selected to identify high-risk individuals most likely to benefit from the cancer-preventive drug. In addition, the use of adaptive clinical trial designs may reduce the number of subjects needed for these studies and thus speed the pace of cancer prevention research.

Secondly, public awareness and sensitivity to possible rare adverse effects occurring from long-term preventive drug use have increased and have made the conduction of clinical cancer prevention trials much more difficult (as was the case with celecoxib and gefitinib). While many of these drugs are tolerated by cancer patients, the potential for even minor side effects becomes a major factor when considering chronic preventive therapy in healthy women. To overcome these problems, future cancer prevention drug development will need to identify effective drugs with minimal toxicity that may be used for short periods or in short pulses. Finally, it will be necessary to educate the public and medical community about the need for risk/benefit analysis when deciding upon cancer-preventive therapy. With a good understanding of the risk and benefits of future cancer-preventive agents, it will be possible to reduce cancer incidence in high-risk individuals who are likely to accept the risk of rare, minor toxicities from effective cancer-preventive drugs.

References

Anzano MA, Byers SW et al (1994) Prevention of breast cancer in the rat with 9-cis-retinoic acid as a single agent and in combination with tamoxifen. Cancer Res 54(17):4614–4617

Ariga R, Zarif A et al (2005) Correlation of her-2/neu gene amplification with other prognostic and predictive factors in female breast carcinoma. Breast J 11(4):278–280

Bailey CJ, Turner RC (1996) Metformin. N Engl J Med 334(9):574–579

Bonovas S, Filioussi K et al (2005) Use of statins and breast cancer: a meta-analysis of seven randomized clinical trials and nine observational studies. J Clin Oncol 23(34):8606–8612

Bryant HE, Schultz N et al (2005) Specific killing of BRCA2-deficient tumours with inhibitors of poly(ADP-ribose) polymerase. Nature 434(7035): 913–917

Campbell MJ, Esserman LJ et al (2006) Breast cancer growth prevention by statins. Cancer Res 66(17):8707–8714

Cazzaniga M, Bonanni B et al (2009) Is it time to test metformin in breast cancer clinical trials? Cancer Epidemiol Biomarkers Prev 18(3):701–705

Chan KC, Knox WF et al (2001) Blockade of growth factor receptors in ductal carcinoma in situ inhibits epithelial proliferation. Br J Surg 88(3): 412–418

Chlebowski R, Cuzick J et al (2009) Clinical perspectives on the utility of aromatase inhibitors for the adjuvant treatment of breast cancer. Breast 18(Suppl 2):S1–11

Clay CE, Namen AM et al (1999) Influence of J series prostaglandins on apoptosis and tumorigenesis of breast cancer cells. Carcinogenesis 20(10):1905–1911

Cummings SR, Eckert S et al (1999) The effect of raloxifene on risk of breast cancer in postmenopausal women: results from the MORE randomized trial. Multiple outcomes of raloxifene evaluation. Jama 281(23):2189–2197

Cummings SR, Ensrud K et al (2010) "Lasofoxifene in postmenopausal women with osteoporosis." N Engl J Med 362(8): 686-96.

Cuzick J (2003). Aromatase inhibitors in prevention – data from the ATAC (arimidex, tamoxifen alone or in combination) trial and the design of IBIS-II (the second International Breast Cancer Intervention Study). Recent Results Cancer Res 163:96–103; discussion 264–266

Cuzick J (2008) IBIS II: a breast cancer prevention trial in postmenopausal women using the aromatase inhibitor anastrozole. Expert Rev Anticancer Ther 8(9):1377–1385

Cuzick J, Baum M (1985) Tamoxifen and contralateral breast cancer. Lancet 2(8449):282

Cuzick J, Forbes JF et al (2007) Long-term results of tamoxifen prophylaxis for breast cancer–96-month follow-up of the randomized IBIS-I trial. J Natl Cancer Inst 99(4):272–282

13

Cuzick J, Powles T et al (2003) Overview of the main outcomes in breast-cancer prevention trials. Lancet 361(9354):296–300

Dannenberg AJ, Lippman SM et al (2005) Cyclooxygenase-2 and epidermal growth factor receptor: pharmacologic targets for chemoprevention. J Clin Oncol 23(2):254–266

Dearth RK, Delgado DA et al (2010) Parity-induced decrease in systemic growth hormone alters mammary gland signaling: A potential role in pregnancy protection from breast cancer. Cancer Preve Res (Phila Pa) 3(3):312–321

Dunn BK, Ryan A (2009) Phase 3 trials of aromatase inhibitors for breast cancer prevention: following in the path of the selective estrogen receptor modulators. Ann N Y Acad Sci 1155:141–161

Fisher B, Costantino JP et al (2005) Tamoxifen for the prevention of breast cancer: current status of the National Surgical Adjuvant Breast and Bowel Project P-1 study. J Natl Cancer Inst 97(22): 1652–1662

Fisher B, Costantino JP et al (1998) Tamoxifen for prevention of breast cancer: report of the National Surgical Adjuvant Breast and Bowel Project P-1 Study. J Natl Cancer Inst 90(18):1371–1388

Fong PC, Boss DS et al (2009) Inhibition of poly(ADP-ribose) polymerase in tumors from BRCA mutation carriers. N Engl J Med 361(2): 123–134

Forbes JF, Cuzick J et al (2008) Effect of anastrozole and tamoxifen as adjuvant treatment for early-stage breast cancer: 100-month analysis of the ATAC trial. Lancet Oncol 9(1):45–53

Garwood ER, Kumar AS et al (2010) "Fluvastatin reduces proliferation and increases apoptosis in women with high grade breast cancer." Breast Cancer Res Treat 119(1): 137-44.

Giardiello FM, Brensinger JD et al (2000) Very high risk of cancer in familial Peutz-Jeghers syndrome. Gastroenterology 119(6):1447–1453

Goodwin PJ (2008) Insulin in the adjuvant breast cancer setting: a novel therapeutic target for lifestyle and pharmacologic interventions? J Clin Oncol 26(6):833–834

Goodwin PJ, Ligibel JA et al (2009) Metformin in breast cancer: time for action. J Clin Oncol 27(20): 3271–3273

Goss PE, Richardson H et al (2007) National Cancer Institute of Canada Clinical Trials Group MAP.3 Trial: evaluation of exemestane to prevent breast cancer in postmenopausal women. Clin Breast Cancer 7(11):895–900

Harris RE, Alshafie GA et al (2000) Chemoprevention of breast cancer in rats by celecoxib, a cyclooxygenase 2 inhibitor. Cancer Res 60(8): 2101–2103

Hong WK, Lippman SM et al (1990) Prevention of second primary tumors with isotretinoin in squamous-cell carcinoma of the head and neck. N Engl J Med 323(12):795–801

Honig SF (2001) Tamoxifen for the reduction in the incidence of breast cancer in women at high risk for breast cancer. Ann N Y Acad Sci 949: 345–348

Horner MJ, Ries LAG, Krapcho M, Neyman N, Aminou R, Howlader N, Altekruse SF, Feuer EJ, Huang L, Mariotto A, Miller BA, Lewis DR, Eisner MP, Stinchcomb DG, Edwards BK (eds) (2009). SEER Cancer Statistics Review, 1975–2006. Retrieved July 15, 2009, 2009, from http://seer.cancer.gov/statfacts/html/breast.html, http://seer.cancer.gov/csr/1975_2006/

Howe LR, Subbaramaiah K et al (2002) Celecoxib, a selective cyclooxygenase 2 inhibitor, protects against human epidermal growth factor receptor 2 (HER-2)/neu-induced breast cancer. Cancer Res 62(19):5405–5407

Hynes NE, Lane HA (2005) ERBB receptors and cancer: the complexity of targeted inhibitors. Nat Rev Cancer 5(5):341–354

Ip MM, Masso-Welch PA et al (1999) Conjugated linoleic acid inhibits proliferation and induces apoptosis of normal rat mammary epithelial cells in primary culture. Exp Cell Res 250(1):22–34

Josefsson ML, Leinster SJ (2010) "Aromatase inhibitors versus tamoxifen as adjuvant hormonal therapy for oestrogen sensitive early breast cancer in postmenopausal women: Meta-analyese of monotherapy, sequenced therapy and extended therapy." Breast.

Khuder SA, Mutgi AB (2001) Breast cancer and NSAID use: a meta-analysis. Br J Cancer 84(9): 1188–1192

Kleinberg DL, Wood TL et al (2009) Growth hormone and insulin-like growth factor-I in the transition from normal mammary development to preneoplastic mammary lesions. Endocr Rev 30(1):51–74

Kong G, Kim HT et al (2005) The retinoid X receptor-selective retinoid, LGD1069, down-regulates cyclooxygenase-2 expression in human breast cells through transcription factor crosstalk: implications for molecular-based chemoprevention. Cancer Res 65(8):3462–3469

Kumar AP, Quake AL et al (2009) Repression of NHE1 expression by PPARgamma activation is a potential new approach for specific inhibition of the growth of tumor cells in vitro and in vivo. Cancer Res 69(22):8636–8644

Kumar AS, Benz CC et al (2008) Estrogen receptor-negative breast cancer is less likely to arise among lipophilic statin users. Cancer Epidemiol Biomarkers Prev 17(5):1028–1033

Kumar AS, Campbell M et al (2006) A call for clinical trials: lipophilic statins may prove effective in treatment and prevention of particular breast cancer subtypes. J Clin Oncol 24(13):2127; author reply 2127–2128

Larsson SC, Mantzoros CS et al (2007) Diabetes mellitus and risk of breast cancer: a meta-analysis. Int J Cancer 121(4):856–862

Lee HY, Dawson MI et al (1996) Retinoic acid receptor- and retinoid X receptor-selective retinoids activate signaling pathways that converge on AP-1 and inhibit squamous differentiation in human bronchial epithelial cells. Cell Growth Differ 7(8):997–1004

Lerner LJ, Holthaus FJ Jr et al (1958) A non-steroidal estrogen antiagonist 1-(p-2-diethylaminoethoxyphenyl)-1-phenyl-2-p-methoxyphenyl ethanol. Endocrinology 63(3):295–318

Li Y, Zhang Y et al (2007) The Rexinoid LG100268 prevents the development of preinvasive and invasive estrogen receptor negative tumors in MMTV-erbB2 mice. Clin Cancer Res 13(20):6224–6231

Liby K, Rendi M et al (2006) The combination of the rexinoid, LG100268, and a selective estrogen receptor modulator, either arzoxifene or acolbifene, synergizes in the prevention and treatment of mammary tumors in an estrogen receptor-negative model of breast cancer. Clin Cancer Res 12(19):5902–5909

Liby K, Risingsong R et al (2008) Prevention and treatment of experimental estrogen receptor-negative mammary carcinogenesis by the synthetic triterpenoid CDDO-methyl Ester and the rexinoid LG100268. Clin Cancer Res 14(14): 4556–4563

Litzenburger BC, Kim HJ et al (2009) BMS-536924 reverses IGF-IR-induced transformation of mammary epithelial cells and causes growth inhibition and polarization of MCF7 cells. Clin Cancer Res 15(1):226–237

Lu C, Speers C et al (2003) Effect of epidermal growth factor receptor inhibitor on development of estrogen receptor-negative mammary tumors. J Natl Cancer Inst 95(24):1825–1833

Maggiora M, Bologna M et al (2004) An overview of the effect of linoleic and conjugated-linoleic acids on the growth of several human tumor cell lines. Int J Cancer 112(6):909–919

Mason RP, Walter MF et al (2004) Effects of HMG-CoA reductase inhibitors on endothelial function: role of microdomains and oxidative stress. Circulation 109(21 Suppl 1):II34–41

Medina D, Kittrell F et al (2009) Prevention of tumorigenesis in p53-null mammary epithelium by rexinoid bexarotene, tyrosine kinase inhibitor gefitinib, and celecoxib. Cancer Prev Res (Phila Pa) 2(2):168–174

Mehta RG, Williamson E et al (2000) A ligand of peroxisome proliferator-activated receptor gamma, retinoids, and prevention of preneoplastic mammary lesions. J Natl Cancer Inst 92(5): 418–423

Moon RC, Thompson HJ et al (1979) N-(4-Hydroxyphenyl)retinamide, a new retinoid for prevention of breast cancer in the rat. Cancer Res 39(4):1339–1346

Moulder SL, Yakes FM et al (2001) Epidermal growth factor receptor (HER1) tyrosine kinase inhibitor ZD1839 (Iressa) inhibits HER2/neu (erbB2)-overexpressing breast cancer cells in vitro and in vivo. Cancer Res 61(24):8887–8895

Mueck AO, Seeger H et al (2003) Effect of statins combined with estradiol on the proliferation of human receptor-positive and receptor-negative breast cancer cells. Menopause 10(4):332–336

Mueller E, Sarraf P et al (1998) Terminal differentiation of human breast cancer through PPAR gamma. Mol Cell 1(3):465–470

Papa V, Belfiore A (1996) Insulin receptors in breast cancer: biological and clinical role. J Endocrinol Invest 19(5):324–333

Powles TJ, Ashley S et al (2007) Twenty-year follow-up of the Royal Marsden randomized, double-blinded tamoxifen breast cancer prevention trial. J Natl Cancer Inst 99(4):283–290

Rendi MH, Suh N et al (2004) The selective estrogen receptor modulator arzoxifene and the rexinoid LG100268 cooperate to promote transforming growth factor beta-dependent apoptosis in breast cancer. Cancer Res 64(10):3566–3571

Rigas B, Kashfi K (2005) Cancer prevention: a new era beyond cyclooxygenase-2. J Pharmacol Exp Ther 314(1):1–8

Salh B, Marotta A et al (1999) Investigation of the Mek-MAP kinase-Rsk pathway in human breast cancer. Anticancer Res 19(1B):731–740

13

Savage DG, Antman KH (2002) Imatinib mesylate–a new oral targeted therapy. N Engl J Med 346(9):683–693

Sawyers CL, Hochhaus A et al (2002) Imatinib induces hematologic and cytogenetic responses in patients with chronic myelogenous leukemia in myeloid blast crisis: results of a phase II study. Blood 99(10):3530–3539

Schreinemachers DM, Everson RB (1994) Aspirin use and lung, colon, and breast cancer incidence in a prospective study. Epidemiology 5(2):138–146

Seewaldt VL, Kim JH et al (1997) All-trans-retinoic acid mediates G1 arrest but not apoptosis of normal human mammary epithelial cells. Cell Growth Differ 8(6):631–641

Shaw RJ, Lamia KA et al (2005) The kinase LKB1 mediates glucose homeostasis in liver and therapeutic effects of metformin. Science 310(5754): 1642–1646

Strecker TE, Shen Q et al (2009) Effect of lapatinib on the development of estrogen receptor-negative mammary tumors in mice. J Natl Cancer Inst 101(2):107–113

Suh N, Wang Y et al (1999) A new ligand for the peroxisome proliferator-activated receptor-gamma (PPAR-gamma), GW7845, inhibits rat mammary carcinogenesis. Cancer Res 59(22): 5671–5673

Szanto A, Narkar V et al (2004) Retinoid X receptors: X-ploring their (patho)physiological functions. Cell Death Differ 11(Suppl 2):S126–143

Turini ME, DuBois RN (2002) Cyclooxygenase-2: a therapeutic target. Annu Rev Med 53:35–57

Tutt A et al (2009) Inhibition of poly(ADP-ribose) polymerase in tumors from BRCA mutation carriers. J Clin Oncol (Suppl) 27(18s): Abstr. CRA501

Uray IP, Shen Q et al (2009) Rexinoid-induced expression of IGFBP-6 requires RARbeta-dependent permissive cooperation of retinoid receptors and AP-1. J Biol Chem 284(1):345–353

Vazquez-Martin A, Oliveras-Ferraros C et al (2009) The antidiabetic drug metformin: a pharmaceutical AMPK activator to overcome breast cancer resistance to HER2 inhibitors while decreasing risk of cardiomyopathy. Ann Oncol 20(3):592–595

Veronesi U, Maisonneuve P et al (2007) Tamoxifen for the prevention of breast cancer: late results of the Italian Randomized Tamoxifen Prevention Trial among women with hysterectomy. J Natl Cancer Inst 99(9):727–737

Vogel VG, Costantino JP et al (2006) Effects of tamoxifen vs raloxifene on the risk of developing invasive breast cancer and other disease outcomes: the NSABP Study of Tamoxifen and Raloxifene (STAR) P-2 trial. JAMA 295(23): 2727–2741

Wendel M, Heller AR (2009) Anticancer actions of omega-3 fatty acids – current state and future perspectives. Anticancer Agents Med Chem 9(4):457–470

Woditschka S, Haag JD et al (2006) Neu-induced retroviral rat mammary carcinogenesis: a novel chemoprevention model for both hormonally responsive and nonresponsive mammary carcinomas. Cancer Res 66(13):6884–6891

Wolbach SB, Howe PR (1925) Tissue changes following deprivation of fat-soluble a vitamin. J Exp Med 42(6):753–777

Wu K, DuPre E et al (2006) Receptor-selective retinoids inhibit the growth of normal and malignant breast cells by inducing G1 cell cycle blockade. Breast Cancer Res Treat 96(2):147–157

Wu K, Kim HT et al (2002a) Suppression of mammary tumorigenesis in transgenic mice by the RXR-selective retinoid, LGD1069. Cancer Epidemiol Biomarkers Prev 11(5):467–474

Wu K, Kim HT et al (2000) 9-cis-Retinoic acid suppresses mammary tumorigenesis in C3(1)-simian virus 40 T antigen-transgenic mice. Clin Cancer Res 6(9):3696–3704

Wu K, Zhang Y et al (2002b) The retinoid X receptor-selective retinoid, LGD1069, prevents the development of estrogen receptor-negative mammary tumors in transgenic mice. Cancer Res 62(22):6376–6380

Xue F, Michels KB (2007) Diabetes, metabolic syndrome, and breast cancer: a review of the current evidence. Am J Clin Nutr 86(3):s823–835

Yang L, Ostrowski J et al (2001) The retinoic acid receptor antagonist, BMS453, inhibits normal breast cell growth by inducing active TGFbeta and causing cell cycle arrest. Oncogene 20(55): 8025–8035

Yin F, Bruemmer D et al (2004) Signaling pathways involved in induction of GADD45 gene expression and apoptosis by troglitazone in human MCF-7 breast carcinoma cells. Oncogene 23(26): 4614–4623

Yin F, Wakino S et al (2001) Troglitazone inhibits growth of MCF-7 breast carcinoma cells by targeting G1 cell cycle regulators. Biochem Biophys Res Commun 286(5):916–922

Zakikhani M, Dowling R et al (2006) Metformin is an AMP kinase-dependent growth inhibitor for breast cancer cells. Cancer Res 66(21): 10269–10273